# Fix My Knee

# Fix My Knee

## A Guide to Preventing and Healing from Injury and Strain

George Demirakos

ROWMAN & LITTLEFIELD
Lanham • Boulder • New York • London

Published by Rowman & Littlefield
A wholly owned subsidiary of The Rowman & Littlefield Publishing Group, Inc.
4501 Forbes Boulevard, Suite 200, Lanham, Maryland 20706
www.rowman.com

Unit A, Whitacre Mews, 26-34 Stannary Street, London SE11 4AB

British Library Cataloguing in Publication Information Available

**Library of Congress Cataloging-in-Publication Data**

Names: Demirakos, George, author.
Title: Fix my knee : a guide to preventing and healing from injury and strain
  / George Demirakos.
Description: Lanham : Rowman & Littlefield, [2018] | Includes bibliographical
  references and index.
Identifiers: LCCN 2017016693 (print) | LCCN 2017018961 (ebook) | ISBN
  9781442211032 (electronic) | ISBN 9781442211025 (cloth : alk. paper)
Subjects: LCSH: Knee. | Knee—Wounds and injuries—Treatment.
Classification: LCC RD561 (ebook) | LCC RD561 .D46 2018 (print) | DDC
  617.5/8044—dc23
LC record available at https://lccn.loc.gov/2017016693

♾™ The paper used in this publication meets the minimum requirements of
American National Standard for Information Sciences—Permanence of Paper
for Printed Library Materials, ANSI/NISO Z39.48-1992.

Printed in the United States of America

# Contents

# Disclaimer

This book represents reference materials only. It is not in any way intended as a medical manual, and the data presented here are meant to assist the reader in making informed choices regarding wellness. This book is not a replacement for treatment(s) that the reader's personal physician may have suggested. If the reader believes he or she is experiencing a medical issue, professional medical help is recommended. Mention of particular products, companies, or authorities in this book does not entail endorsement by the publisher or author.

The first step that should be taken is to speak to your doctor before beginning any exercise program.

Even a minor knee injury, unevaluated and untreated by a professional, can lead to decreasing or eliminating the normal function of the knee. Don't wait; please get professional help today!

# Acknowledgments

It is very rare for one to get an opportunity to write a book that they dream of writing, let alone a second one. I am so deeply blessed and express my immense gratitude to all the individuals who have guided me and to those whom I never met helping me to go down this road again and to write this book. To all of you who continue to cheer me on, thank you very much.

To Sarah Jane Freymann, my incredible book agent, who brought me under her wing and helped me grow: thank you for everything.

To my publishing company, Rowman & Littlefield, as well as to my uber-talented and special editor, Suzanne Staszak-Silva: working with you has been an absolute pleasure, and thank you once again for making my dreams and passions come true!

I would also like to thank Caitlin Bean, Erin McGarvey, Will True, and the amazing staff at Rowman & Littlefield who work tirelessly to turn my work into magic.

Thanks also to Alan Michael Wong, for being a wizard with the camera and for the amazing pictures.

Family is everything, so I would like to thank my mom and dad, as well as my awesome sisters for supporting me throughout this process. They always tell me to do everything with a smile.

I would also like to extend a special thank-you to my in-laws, Nunzio and Maria, and my brothers-in-law, Tony and Mike, for always being there for me and my family. They are always giving and never ask for anything in return. I am very lucky to have an extended family like you guys on my side. *Mille grazie!*

For their expert advice and valuable therapeutic knowledge that was shared with me, I thank the following teachers: Dr. David Paris, Scott Livingston, Ron Rappel, Dave Campbell, as well as the late Edith Aston-McCrimmon.

Some personal shout-outs to the following amazing people who, in their own special ways, have given me the insane drive and uplifting inspiration to write this book: Mr. Dwayne Johnson, Miss Jillian Michaels, Mr. John Cena, and Mr. Gordon Ramsay. You guys are awesome!

There are some very special people who work in the Hearst Building where the incredible *O* and *Redbook* magazines are created. They opened their doors and hearts to me and made me feel like a part of their family. A special thank-you goes out to Miss Gayle King, Miss Jayne Jamison, and Mr. Ron Balasco from the *O* magazine family, as well as to Miss Wendi Cassuto and staff from the *Redbook* family, who made our day one that we will never forget!

A big high five to those special runners who have inspired me to take up the sport. Thank you to Debbie, M. C., and my other runner patients, to whom the running chapter is dedicated. A shout-out to all the amazing staff at the Running Room, who love what they do and are amazing at it!

A sincere thank-you goes out to all my patients who, over the years, have trusted me with helping them treat their knee injuries. I hope you enjoy reading this book as much as I enjoyed writing it.

To my special kids, Michael-Anthony and Kayla, thank you for always letting daddy run down to the basement to write his book and not play with you guys every day. I love you both so very much, and I am the luckiest guy in the world to have you both in my life. You put a smile on my face every day.

Lastly, I would like to thank my wife, Frankie. Without you, I can't do what I do. This book is dedicated to you. You are the reason that I can write, I can love, and I can live. Your daily encouragement made me believe that I can do anything, even if I didn't want to believe it myself. Thank you for being my best friend. I love you.

# Introduction

All successes begin with self-discipline. It starts with you.

—Dwayne Johnson

Vincent loves computers. From the time he was a young boy working in his father's shop, he loved taking computers apart, piece by piece, and putting them back together again. The anatomy of this machine was easy for him to understand. He was well versed in modems, hard drives, Wi-Fi, and the like. He was also a great basketball player, nicknamed "ankle tripper" by his teammates for the huge thud his opponents made when they hit the ground, tripping over their ankles, trying to keep up with his lighting speed and quick cuts to the basket. However, when Vincent's doctor advised him that his constant knee pain was a result of a partial MCL strain, he was clueless about how an important part of his own anatomy—a ligament that was attached to two bones—was turning his world upside down. He secretly wished that he could zip around this problem as fast as he could zip around the basketball court.

Knee injuries are one of the most common joint problems of the body, next to neck and back pain, and knees are by far the most common site of pain and disability in a person's arms and legs. Individuals between the ages of fifteen to twenty-nine have the highest incidence of injuries.

Whether you're focused on long-distance running, sports that require plenty of cutting and sharp lateral movement, heavy lifting, or any sort of strenuous activity that's hard on the legs, the well-being of your knees and the muscles around them is an essential part of your fitness goals, even if keeping them strong and supple isn't necessarily part of your program.

For most, knee injuries seem to happen suddenly, or they creep up over time. However, there are definite things all athletes and fitness devotees can do to prevent knee problems from occurring. That comes from really listening and respecting your body and not doing too much at any given time, while also knowing which muscles to strengthen so that your knees and legs are kept in working order.

The truth is that even if you've never felt any kind of knee pain whatsoever, the chances are good that as you grow older, you will. Our bodies tend to lose muscle and bone mass as we age, and we become more susceptible to the aches and pains that may result.

When we injure the knee in some way, it naturally stops working as it should. It won't bend fully or pull quite as forcefully. That makes it hard to pick something up from the floor or to pull something down from overhead. Spending hours in front of the computer becomes torture. Lifting groceries out of the car and carrying them into the house becomes an ordeal. New grandparents can't stand up comfortably to hold their grandbaby.

But neither weakness nor pain is inevitable. The knee can be fixed, and the pain can go away. First, there's a systematic way to cure the weakness and end the pain. But there's also a way that can help to prevent the problem to begin with so that you never lose the strength, stability, and range of motion of the knee at all. I can show you both, and that is what I do in *Fix My Knee.*

## GETTING A CLEAR SENSE OF WHAT REALLY IS GOING ON

When people think of the knee joint, they usually think of the tibia, femur, and patella, or kneecap; they often see it as a hinge joint that bends and straightens. When these bones are healthy, they slide on each other really well. But when there is damage to the cartilage on the bone, it can start to create damage on the bone, and, therefore, the joint won't work as well as it used to.

Adding to the problem is any sort of weakness in the surrounding muscles around the knee, and that, too, can create the starting point of knee troubles. Getting your knees healthier is therefore first and foremost about balancing the strength of the muscles of the knee as well as having optimal flexibility. This is also important for preventing knee troubles in the first place.

## Why a Book about the Knee?

There is a lot of information out there. Most people would just Google the question in hopes of finding the information that they are looking for. The problem is that you do not know if what you are getting is based upon peer-documented research that has been accepted by the medical community or by individuals who "believe" that they can help you because they have a similar problem. That is not always the case. The information in this book is based upon my years of expertise as a practicing physical therapist, as well as documented research. It also was written to help set you on the right path to healing your knee.

Now, please let me make myself perfectly clear. There most definitely will be lots of cases and situations in which your knee problem must be seen and treated by a medical professional, such as your physician and your physical therapist, and you should definitely go for the necessary treatment sessions required by your therapist. One of the reasons that I am writing this book is to help guide those who have straightforward, simple issues with their knees. With a little guidance from my recommendations and suggestions—like a good, balanced exercise program that readers can follow at home—I can save them some time, money, and significant discomfort. I also believe in educating readers so that some of the issues that might be confusing at first can become clear.

This book is primarily written for individuals with knee pain that appeared out of the blue, with no apparent cause, and that has been bothering them on and off for a while. I hope it also helps people who, despite seeing a gamut of professionals, were left with no real hope for alleviating their pain. I don't believe in a completely different knee program for a weekend warrior playing soccer, for example, and for a runner training for a 5K. We all have the same anatomy, and the pain, range of motion, and strength rules are for every person regardless of age, race, gender, or socioeconomic status. Therefore we all fall under the same category. I believe that the only thing that distinguishes an athlete from an everyday individual is perhaps the sophisticated equipment at their disposal or the specific, higher-level exercises that help them attain the highest level in their specific sport.

Sometimes when people visit me at the clinic, they are surprised when I tell them that the most important component that will help relieve their pain and discomfort are exercises that can be done at home. In some instances, just a few very specific exercises. No one will do hours of daily exercises, no matter how great his or her pain. Patients are surprised; they

believe that because the pain is so great, it must require a more complicated treatment than a home exercise program. They are sceptical that
exercises really could help them.[1] Every knee problem does not require
surgical intervention and an exercise program can help.

So, what topics are going to be covered in this book? In chapter 1, titled
"The Knee Blueprint," we look at the way our knee is put together with all
of its relative anatomy. It is interesting to note that our knee—although
made of bones, muscles, ligaments, just like our shoulder—works a little
differently. Our shoulder, being a ball-and-socket joint, has a wide range
of motion. We can make circles with our arms, no problem; our knee,
however, is a hinge joint. Its primary movements are front and back, and
it does not have many degrees of freedom. Whereas a shoulder is very
flexible but not very stable, and requiring the rotator muscles to stabilize
the joint, a knee is the opposite. It is very stable and strong, but the flexibility of the muscles around it might need some work. This is why some
people hate stretching.

Chapter 2 looks at some of the things that can go wrong with the knee.
We examine the differences between male and female knee pain and why
they are different, as well as discuss different types of knee injuries. What
is tendinitis, and how does it differ from bursitis? What about house-
maid knee versus tennis knee? There are all sorts of different conditions,
and hopefully we can demystify some of them. This chapter specifically
addresses why and how things can go wrong, producing the kind of de-
bilitating pain and discomfort that causes readers to seek out this book,
enabling and empowering them with precisely that understanding.

The title of chapter 3 comes from a saying that I sometimes hear from
my patients: "My knee is shot! Get me a new one!" I discuss different
types of pain and why it happens. Most people say that their pain "came
out of nowhere suddenly," but we see that it's not necessarily the case. I
show you how to tell the difference between a traumatic and biomechanical injury. I'll also lay out the first steps to take when you feel pain—like
how to reduce inflammation or rest an overused tendon. The last thing
you want to do is make the condition worse. Chapter 3 ensures that you
don't do that, so you can begin the healing of your knee quickly, confidently, and effectively. It also answers the question that is on everyone's
mind: Should I put ice or heat on it?

Chapter 4 is everyone's favorite chapter. Here, I show you the exercises
that can help you get your knee feeling better, stronger, and more supple
than ever before. This is where I show you the different types of exercises

that you can do, how many, and how often. I also cover mistakes that you should look out for so that you do not hurt yourself further. I offer some diverse range-of-motion and strength routines, ranging from very simple and basic to more advanced versions. I explain the purpose of every exercise so that you get a clear understanding of why you are doing it—not just because your physio told you to. I hope these routines make you feel confident in accomplishing your everyday tasks, as well as in participating in the sport that you love.

Chapter 5 focuses on running, a sport practiced by more than sixty million people in the United States alone. We look at ways to run and how to stretch and train better in order to run more efficiently, use less energy, and balance your muscle strength so that you can move better. I also talk about proper shoes to wear while running and why foot strength might be the biggest weak link in the body, as well as why "rolling" might not be as effective as people might think. I promise that these techniques will make readers feel as good as new after a long day! I provide as much information as I can so that your doctor never tells you to stop running. I prepare you to run.

Finally, in chapter 6, "Getting Your Knee into Super Shape," I cover the prevention program of exercises that you can do in your gym or at home to develop the strength, flexibility, and coordination that you need to participate in any sport, recreational activity, or just everyday life with the confidence and assuredness that you want. I create some exercise routines for your favorite sports and get you ready to have fun!

Although this book has been written to be read from the beginning to the end, I also suggest and encourage you to use it as a reference tool, referring to the parts that specifically pertain to you. Bring it, if you like, to your doctor appointment. By using the information contained here, you can speed up your understanding of your knee pain, thus making your game plan that much easier to implement.

I truly hope that you find this book entertaining and informative. I wrote it to help people with knee problems who want answers to their questions. I am a physiotherapist by occupation, and I love my job. I love helping people, and I hope, in some way, this book helps to relieve your knee pain and improve your quality of life.

I hope you enjoy reading this book as much as I did writing it.

# 1

# The Knee Blueprint

Impossible is temporary: Impossible is nothing

—Muhammad Ali

Your knee can do a lot of things that you don't realize. You might crouch down to pick up your child, or you might run full tilt to catch that bus. You might climb a flight of stairs or jump over a pothole you saw at the last minute. Perhaps we take our knees for granted, thinking they will obey us forever. But the more we use our knees—whether for daily sports or for everyday chores—the more wear and tear develops. Like any type of equipment, they could break down at some point. We need to have a basic understanding of all the parts of the knee joint and of what is involved in its movement and function. When we know what parts make up our knee and how they move, we can do the necessary strengthening and stretching exercises needed to keep our body humming along and prevent it from breaking down, keeping both your mind and body in good health.

Just think: millions of people from weekend warriors to Olympic athletes play at their highest levels, participating in the sports that they love at full force, and yet they don't get injured. There must be a reason for that. The secret to the knee's amazing variability and power lies in the way it was created. Its anatomical design is truly ingenious. So let's take a look at how our knees are put together.

## THE BONES OF THE KNEE

Did you know that the knee is the largest joint in the human body? The three bones that meet to form the knee is the thighbone, called the femur; the shinbone, referred to as the tibia; and the patella, which is the kneecap. There is also a fourth bone found on the outside part of the tibia called the fibula. These bones are what we call static stabilizers, and their job is to provide structure and stability. Much like the foundation of a house, static stabilizers are your body's foundation.

First off, you have your femur bone. It is the longest bone of your body. The femur makes up approximately 25 percent of a person's height and is considered the strongest bone in your body. It takes an incredible amount of force to break it. The number-one cause of a femur break or fracture is car accidents. The top part of the femur, or the head, connects directly into your pelvis, creating your hip joint. The bottom part of the femur connects with the tibia and kneecap to create your knee joint. It is the only bone in the thigh, and it is used as an attachment point for all of the muscles that contract and use their force over the hip and knee joints. There are also some muscles that cross two joints, called the biarticular joints, such as the gastrocnemius, or calf muscle, and the plantaris muscle, which start at the femur. In total, there are twenty-two muscles that either start from or connect to the femur.

The bone that lies beneath the femur is called the tibia. The bone next to it is the fibula. The tibia is the larger and stronger of these two bones. The tibia is made up of three parts: the shaft in the middle and the two round extremities called the epiphysis and diaphysis. The tibia is the second largest bone in the body next to the femur. It is so strong that it can withstand the force placed from the top of the bone to the bottom, called axial placed force, during walking, which is up to approximately five times a person's actual bodyweight. Whereas the tibia is the powerhouse and absorbs most of your bodyweight, the fibula is the opposite: it barely absorbs any weight at all. The fibula has a head and neck, as well as an anterior and posterior border. It connects to the back of the head of the tibia; therefore, it is not part of the knee joint. The fibula forms the outer part of the ankle, creating stability for this joint. Many ligaments attach to the fibula, which gives them leverage and helps the muscles produce their force. It also provides muscular attachment and functions to support the tibia.

Last, we come to the kneecap, or patella. The word *patella* originated in the seventeenth century and derives from the Latin word *patina*, which means "shallow dish." Looks like one, doesn't it? It is a thick, triangular bone that articulates with the femur and covers and protects the anterior area of the knee joint. It is the largest sesamoid bone in the body. A sesamoid bone is a bone that is embedded or found inside the tendon or muscle; in this case, the patella is embedded in the quadriceps tendon. The lowest part of the patella is pointy, and this is where the patella tendon originates. Its primary function is to help extend the knee. Due to the way the patella is connected to the patellar tendon, the patella can increase the leverage that the tendon exerts on the femur by increasing the angle that it acts on. That's why you get a smooth action and movement of your kneecap when you extend you knee. The patella is stabilized by fibers of the vastus medialis muscle of your quadriceps, which I talk about a little later, as well as the lateral condyle of your femur.

## THE JOINTS OF THE KNEE

The knee joint is a hinge joint. It moves like a hinge: primarily back and forth with a little bit of medial and lateral rotation. The joints are created by a spongy cushioning surface made of cartilage found at the end of each bone, which protects the ends of the bones by absorbing shock from impact. It also helps to prevent rubbing of the bones. It looks like shiny marble that you might walk on. Shiny, but very strong. When this cartilage gets damaged due to excessive rubbing, it is called arthritis, which I discuss later.

The tibiofemoral joint is the first main joint of the knee, comprising the medial and lateral sides, or condyles, of the femur, which connect to the tibia. The tibiofemoral joint is the weight-bearing joint of the knee. The patellofemoral joint is made of the femur bone connecting to the articulating surfaces of the patella. The patella is found inside the tendon of the quadriceps muscle; its function is to help reduce wear and tear on the tendon. The patellofemoral joint allows the tendon of the quadriceps muscle, which is the main extensor of the knee, to be inserted directly over the knee, increasing the efficiency of the muscle. The third joint, which is the tibiofibular joint, is where the fibula connects to the tibia with ligaments. There is a superior tibiofibular joint, which is related to the knee, and the inferior tibiofibular joint, which is related to the ankle.

## THE BURSAS OF THE KNEE

Before discussing the many bursas around the knee, let's talk about what a bursa is: a fluid-filled sac or structure whose primary purpose is to reduce friction between two moving structures. It is normally found between skin and tendon or tendon and bone. Irritation or inflammation of this structure is called bursitis. There are eleven bursas in the knee. Bursas of the knee are grouped in two areas: those around the patella and those that are not. The patellar bursas include the prepatellar bursa—the bursa in front of the kneecap—and the suprapatellar and infrapatellar bursas, which are above and below the kneecap. The pes anserine bursa is found between the tibia and the hamstring muscle. The hamstring muscle is located behind the femur. It provides a cushion for motion that occurs between the hamstring tendons and the medial collateral ligament (MCL). This ligament can be found underneath the semitendinosus tendon of the hamstring.

## THE MENISCI OF THE KNEE

The word *meniscus* (or menisci, plural) comes from the Greek word meaning "crescent." The two menisci of the knee are made of cartilage and are both a half-moon shape. Their purpose is to disperse the weight of the body, as well as to reduce friction as the body is moving. They are known as the "shock absorbers" of your knee. They essentially spread the load of the body's weight through movement. When you land after jumping, the meniscus's job is to cushion the impact. The lateral meniscus, found on the outer part of the knee joint, is not directly connected to the lateral collateral ligament (LCL). The medial meniscus, however, is directly connected to the anterior cruciate ligament (ACL), as well as the MCL, the ligament that we spoke about earlier. Due to the knee's anatomy, more injuries occur to the medial meniscus, the ACL, and the MCL than to the lateral meniscus.

## THE LIGAMENTS OF THE KNEE

Bones are connected to each other by ligaments, which are made by cartilage. In the knee, there are four major ligaments that help stabilize the knee. Although they can stretch a little bit, they are designed to keep the bones together to protect your leg from going too far out of alignment by stopping your movement in all four directions. It allows your knee to move but not too much.

Two ligaments are found on either side of your leg. As mentioned before, your LCL is on the outside of your leg and is sometimes referred to as the fibular collateral ligament. It is not connected to either the lateral meniscus or the capsule of the knee. This is why there are fewer injuries to the LCL than to the MCL. The MCL is located on the inner part of your leg. Because it connects with the ACL and the medial meniscus, when force gets applied to this area, more injuries can occur. The purpose of both of these ligaments is to stop the left and right forces, or the valgus and varus forces, on the knee. Basically, this prevents the knee from moving side to side.

The other two ligaments stop movements from going front to back too much. The posterior cruciate ligament (PCL) is a tough ligament that is larger and stronger than the ACL. PCL injuries make up about 20 percent

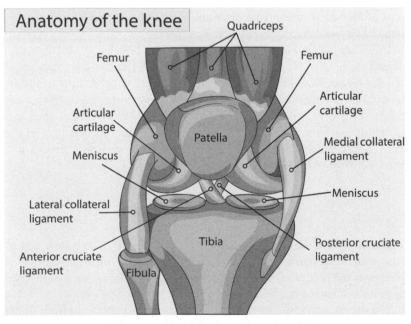

Anatomy of the Knee. *Toricheks, image from Bigstockphoto.com*

of knee ligament injuries, and when the PCL is damaged, usually another ligament or structure is also damaged along with it. The infamous ACL is one of the most commonly injured ligaments of the entire knee complex. It prevents the tibia bone from sliding out in front of the femur bone, stopping overextension of the knee. If your leg goes backward and you were not born like that, it would be a good time to go see a health specialist. The ACL also stabilizes the knee during rotational movements.

## THE TENDONS OF THE KNEE

Tendons are a continuation of muscles, and they help support stability as they expand and contract with movement. As mentioned before, a ligament connects a bone to another bone, and a tendon connects a muscle to a bone. For example, the quadriceps tendon brings all the parts of the quadriceps muscle together and attaches itself onto the upper part of the patella. It then becomes the patellar tendon; the lower part connects to the tibia bone below. The hamstring tendons run on the back of the knee on the medial, or inner, side as well as the lateral, or outer, side. The quadriceps tendon helps the quadriceps muscle extend the leg as the hamstring tendons help the hamstring muscle flex the leg.

One note about a tissue called the iliotibial (IT) band, which is discussed frequently, especially among runners. The IT band is made up of fibrous tissue. The IT band is wide and long, unlike other thin and short tendons, and connects from the outside of your outer thigh, all the way down to the tibia, where it attaches. Its function is to extend, adduct, and laterally rotate the hip. It also helps to stabilize the outside part of the knee. Because it stabilizes the knee in extension and partial flexion, it is used a great deal during walking and running.

## THE MUSCLES OF THE KNEE

The muscles are the movers and shakers of the knee. They allow you to run, jump, slow down, and speed up. They also allow for rotation or stopping and starting. The muscles surrounding your knee are some of the largest muscles in your body.

The quadriceps muscle is a group of four muscles found in front of the femur bone. The word *quadriceps* is Latin for "four headed." The four muscles are: the vastus lateralis, the vastus medialis, the vastus interme-dius, and the rectus femoris. The quadriceps starts at the top of the femur and connects to the tibia, with the exception of the rectus femoris, which starts from the pelvis, crosses the hip area, and attaches to the tibia. The main function of the quadriceps, or quads for short, is very important: the extension of the knee. This is important because extending the knee is the movement required to walk, run, climb stairs, and a lot of other functions that we take for granted. In addition to knee extension, the rectus femoris also flexes the hip upward. Another important function of the quadriceps, specifically the vastus medialis, is stabilizing the patella and the knee joint when you are walking. I believe that when this muscle weakens, it de-creases the stability of the patella, allowing it to become loose and to start rubbing against the cartilage of the femur, which causes those popping and crackling noises that you might hear. It is the sound that grandma makes when she is coming down the stairs in the morning. She might not have the proper balance of strength among the muscles in her knees.

The hamstrings muscles are often neglected muscles compared to their star cousins, the quadriceps. Hamstrings are found in the back of the leg. They are made up of the semimembranosus, semitendinosus, and the outermost muscle, the bicep femoris. They start from underneath your backside (on your sit bones) and attach to the inside and outside parts of the knee just below the joint line. The hamstrings are unique because they pass through two joints: the hips as well as the knee. Therefore they play an important role in the process of walking, jumping, running, as well as help in working together with your quadriceps muscle to decelerate your knee extension. One of the most common knee problems results from hamstrings that are too tight or weak in comparison to the quadriceps. This is discussed extensively later.

Another group of muscles located on the inner part of the leg is called the adductor muscles. There are the short adductor muscles—called the pectineus, adductor longus, and adductor brevis—as well as the long ad-ductor muscles, called the gracilis and adductor magnus. These muscles serve many different functions depending on the specific muscle, but what they all have in common is movement—adduction. Adduction means moving the leg in the direction of the center of the body. Another way you can think about it is moving your straight leg toward your other leg. I find that the adductor muscles are often neglected in training in favor of the abductor muscles, which push the leg out and away from the midline of the body (i.e., away from the other leg). Abduction is a movement that we do often; in running, for example. We move our leg forward, then abduct or swing it away from body, then extend it to the back, then bring it back in front. We don't really bring our leg to the middle. Abduction is even more prevalent in skating or rollerblading, where we push our leg away, then bring it to the middle, then push away again. This is why most hockey players, runners, and even cyclists have strong and tight muscles on the outside of their thighs; compared to the strength and power of the adductors on the inside of the leg, there is quite a bit of a difference. It is said that avoiding injuries is about being balanced. Weak and tight adductor muscles result in groin strain and knee pain, which can prevent you from playing sports or performing some of the basic functions of everyday life.

Another muscle group that I believe is important to talk about here are the gluteal muscles. Yes, the ones that you sit on! The three main glute muscles are the gluteus maximus (or the shorter version, called the bum!), the gluteus medius, and the gluteus minimus. One of their most important functions is to stop or counteract gravity's pull and to turn your knee inward and toward your other leg, or to the midline of your body. They help maintain your body's proper leg alignment through eccentric movement; for example, bending down to tie a shoe or going down stairs. Due to our sedentary lifestyle, we lose tone and strength in our glutes, causing a delay in activation of these muscles, eventually causing them to atrophy. I believe that a good strengthening knee program involves strengthening the glute muscles.

## PROPRIOCEPTIVE NEUROMUSCULAR CONTROL OF THE KNEE

Having great strength and flexibility is important, but if you don't have your muscles and other structures working in unison—firing when they need to fire and being silent when other areas are working—then nothing will work properly, and that will lead to injuries. It has been shown in studies that balance and proprioception of the knee is lost after an injury and must be regained if the individual—weekend warrior or professional athlete—wants to get back to the sport he or she loves. The combination of nerves and muscles that work together with the spinal cord and the brain gives your legs, and especially your knees, that fine-tuning they deserve to help you do the things in life that you love most, whether jogging or running after your kids. Balance and proprioception also keep your knees healthy for life.

## MOTHER NATURE'S SPECIAL LIQUID FOR THE KNEE

The liquid found in the knee is called synovial fluid. It is found in the capsule of knee, which is a saclike structure that surrounds the knee. This thick liquid helps lubricate and reduce friction on all articular joint surfaces, allowing them to move smoothly, kind of like what WD-40 does to creaky door hinges. The fluid is also known as a nutrient transporter, bringing food and oxygen to the cartilage around the knee and removing carbon dioxide and other waste products. This is why exercises are so

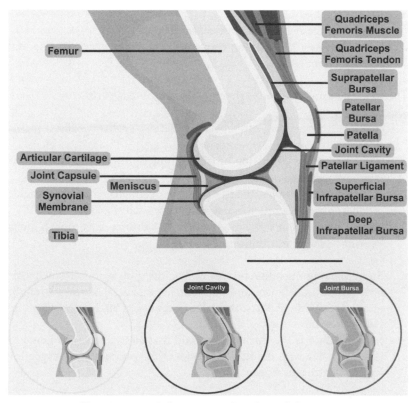

Knee Anatomy. *Lukaves, image from Bigstockphoto.com*

important: movement pumps the synovial fluid into the area, nourishing the cartilage. Why is that so important? What would happen if there was little or no synovial fluid? When there is no lubricant in the knee, arthritis, specifically osteoarthritis, starts to develop.

## SUMMARY

- The four major bones of the knee are the femur, or thigh bone; the tibia, or shin bone; the fibula, which works together with the tibia; and the kneecap, or patella bone.
- The three joints of the knee are the tibiofemoral joint, which joins the femur and tibia; the tib-fib joint, which joins the tibia to the fibula; and the patellofemoral joint, which is considered the largest joint in the body.
- The main ligaments of the knee are the ACL, PCL, MCL, and LCL. They join bone to bone and prevent the leg from veering off in any one direction.

The four main muscle groups that work with the knee are:

1. the quads, consisting of the vastus lateralis, vastus medialis, vastus intermedius, and rectus femoris;
2. the hamstrings, consisting of the semimembranosus, semitendinosus, and biceps femoris;
3. the adductor muscles, made up of the pectineus, adductor longus, adductor brevis, adductor magnus, and gracilis;
4. and the gluteal muscles, made up of the gluteus maximus, gluteus medius, and gluteus minimus.

- Strengthening the adductors as well as the gluteal muscles helps alleviate knee imbalances and decrease knee pain. Balancing strength and flexibility in all parts of the leg and knee is vital to long-lasting, pain-free knees.
- Synovial fluid is the thick, shiny fluid that allows bones in joints to slide and glide with fluidity. It provides nourishment and oxygen for the cartilage of the knee.

# 2

# Why Is Your Knee
# at Risk for Injury?

I love heels, I'm telling you. When I walk in flats, I get knee pain.

—Sofia Vergara

Knee pain can be scary. One day, you're walking up a flight of stairs, wondering what you'll have for lunch, or walking the dog around the block, when out of nowhere, you get this stabbing pain on the inside of your leg. You might end up hobbling to your desk or back home and start asking your neighbors or colleagues if they ever experienced the type of knee pain that you have. Although they mean well, they may tell you that you have arthritis or that a neighbor had the same pain and had to undergo surgery. Maybe you look it up on the Internet, and after a few minutes, you wish you hadn't done that. Another sleepless night full of fear and apprehension forces you to the emergency room. It is always an advantage to know some of the most common injuries of the knee. Understanding what some of the conditions actually mean and why they are associated with the knee gives you a clearer comprehension of what your doctor, therapist, or allied health professional tells you.

Some of the risk factors associated with knee pain follow.

## AGE

The most common risk factor associated with knee pain is age. The older you get, the more wear and tear on your knees. If left untreated, joints can degenerate, which is commonly called osteoarthritis. It normally begins at age fifty for most people, and it can cause pain, stiffness, and inflammation of the knees. It is also important to point out that it is not just older people who have knee pain. Children, who are still growing, have loose parts as they are maturing. They can have fractures and dislocations of the knees because they have not reached maturity, as the muscles and soft tissue that protect the knee have to catch up to the bones.

## GENDER

Every kid loves to play. Whether you are a boy or girl, we are all the same when it comes to playing sports or other fun games. However, boys and girls are different in the way they are made. Although boys and girls basically have the same leg strength until puberty, recent research by Holm and Vollestad demonstrates something different.[1] It states that there is a significant difference between the strength of girls' quadriceps to their hamstring—called the hamstring/quadriceps (HQ) ratios—compared with boys' HQ ratios, as well as the static balance in children between ages eight and twelve. The boys demonstrated significantly higher HQ ratios than the girls in every age group. This means that the hamstring muscle strength in girls is weaker when compared to their quadriceps muscles. This is significant: because a girl's quadriceps are stronger than her hamstrings, different forces act on her knees relative to boys of the same age. Boys had a better balance of strength between their quadriceps and hamstring muscles. The study also shows that girls have much better balance than boys. When puberty hits, the imbalances are even more pronounced. A girl's hips get wider, which means that her "Q-angle" gets wider. The Q angle of the knee is a measurement of the angle between the quadriceps muscles and the patella tendon that gives us information about the alignment of the knee joint. The normal Q angle for a male is 14 degrees, whereas for a female it is 17 degrees due to naturally wider hips. A bigger Q angle can cause abnormal tracking of the kneecap or patella in the space or groove of the femur, where the patella is supposed to pass through. As a result, it has been shown that activities that involve the quadriceps place a different torque on the anterior cruciate ligament (ACL) than it would for boys the same age. Mountcastle and his colleagues at Duke University found that female gymnasts are more than five times as likely to injure their knees compared with male gymnasts, as well as more than two times more likely to rupture their ACL compared with boys playing basketball.

A research paper by Gilchrist and Al, published in the *American Journal of Sports Medicine*, questioned whether female athletes should warm up differently from their male counterparts. They determined that instead of running or performing jumping jacks like the traditional warm-up regime advocated by coaches throughout the years, women should definitely train differently. Because girls' hamstrings are weaker than their quads, an exercise program that includes hamstring curls and running backward stimulates the hamstring and glute strength, and side-to-side jumps improves the balance of strength with their quads. You don't need any special equipment to do this. It has been shown that this type of training—focusing on hamstring strength—decreases the risk of noncontact ACL injury by almost 70 percent compared with girls performing the traditional warm-ups that boys do. Focusing on efficiency makes a significant difference, and if coaches and the players themselves understand and apply this, injuries to girls will decrease dramatically, I believe.

Another issue with the wider pelvis and greater Q angle that girls develop when they reach puberty is that their knees buckle inward, and they stand more upright when landing a jump. Also, when female athletes "cut," or suddenly change direction when running, she will probably do it on one leg, unlike male athletes who would probably perform the same movement with both legs. This is again due to the wider pelvis. Women are also more flexible due to their looser ligaments, and that can create less stability. Therefore, muscle training and strengthening is key. When women focus on training their hamstrings and glutes, as well as strengthening their vastus medialis (the inner part of the quadriceps), it greatly decreases ACL and patellofemoral injuries, therefore keeping them strong. Another component that women can focus on is their balance and proprioception. Proprioception, or knowing where your body is in space—specifically the sensation of one's limbs and trunk—allows your body to work in concert like a fine-tuned orchestra. For example, this allows us to walk in the dark without losing our balance or tell the difference between the brake and the accelerator while driving a car. Injury to muscles and ligaments definitely decrease balance and proprioception. Proprioception can be trained (actually retrained) to keep your knees, ankles, and limbs strong and supple, ultimately keeping them healthy.

Don't get me wrong: balance training is not just for the athletes; it is for everyone, from the weekend warrior to the elderly. Balance training is instrumental in reducing falls in older adults with balance problems and women with weak bone density. It also helps with postural stability, especially after suffering a stroke.

Balance might be a little more complicated than you might realize: the body relies on input from several of its systems, which include the eyes and vestibular system.

## Eyes

This is a no-brainer, but to understand how important your vision is for balance, see if you can stand on one leg with your eyes closed for thirty seconds. (Please make sure that there is a chair or bed beside you, so that you don't fall on your head.) If you are wobbly or jumping around everywhere, don't worry; balance training can help stabilize you. Our eyes also help us adjust our body's position, so we can move around obstacles that might be in our way.

## Vestibular System

If you've ever suffered from vertigo or dizziness, you probably know that balance problems can be created by inner ear trouble. Small nerve receptors—the utricle and the saccule—in the semicircular canals that are part of your inner ear are sensitive to movement of the head, and they relay the position of the body to the brain.

## PROPRIOCEPTION

Small receptors called proprioceptors, which are found in your skin, joints, ligaments, tendons, and muscles, receive stimuli—for example, pressure on the bottoms of the feet—indicating the position, orientation, and movement of your body and send that information to your brain. Your brain then uses that information to create a constantly changing map of your position in space. When you lift your right leg, for example, the map is updated, and you maintain your balance by unconsciously shifting your body weight to your left leg.

You need sensory input, fine motor control, as well as muscle power to maintain stability during both everyday movements, such as lifting a foot off the ground during an exercise routine, and movements that demand reflex, such as recovery from a sudden stumble to avoid falling down. Injury, illness, neurological disorders, certain medications, as well as advancing age can affect all the systems involved in balance, which is why it should always be part of your training regime.

## WEIGHT

This is something that I think everyone knows about, but I want to get into the specifics of why too much weight can hurt your knees. According to the latest statistics, more than a third (36.5 percent) of adults living in the United States are obese. Anyone with a BMI (body mass index) greater than 30 is considered obese. A word of caution: BMI should be used as a *guide*. A very muscular person may have a high BMI because muscle weighs more than fat. You should consult your doctor if you have concerns.

Being overweight can have severe consequences on the health of your knee. Your body frame can support only so much weight. When you exceed that weight, your body is bearing a weight for which it simply was not designed. Excess weight stresses the areas that hold you up, like your ankles, knees, hips, and back. Losing that excessive weight takes pressure off your knees, and fewer injuries will occur because of it. According to research published in the *Journal of Pain Research*, researchers Zdziarski and colleagues stated that people with a BMI greater than 30 have four times the risk of developing osteoarthritis than those who are at a healthy weight.[2] Every pound of excess body weight puts approximately five pounds of pressure on your knee, so even five to ten extra pounds places a burden on you. Maintaining an appropriate weight is one of the best things that you can do for your knee and overall health. It is beyond the scope of this book to offer advice on how to lose weight, but your medical doctor and a nutritionist are good places to start. I'm sure some of you might be thinking, "but every time I exercise, my knees hurt." I completely understand this, and there are ways around it. You can start with something easier than a treadmill. Swimming or even starting on a stationary bike are two great ways that you can get the ball rolling. Start with a little exercise, and gradually build up your endurance. In no time, you'll start to feel stronger and you'll want to train more and more.

## FLEXIBILITY

Everybody hates stretching. Stretching always goes on the back burner, no matter if you're a weekend warrior, an Olympic athlete marathoner, or a professional athlete making millions every year. Why should we do it, and is it necessary? If you want to protect yourself from knee injuries, then it is a good idea to stay flexible. You always want to have at least three elements in a joint: strength, balance, and range of motion. You can acquire strength and balance through strength and proprioception exercises, but to improve range of motion, especially around the joint, stretching is a must. When you have a greater range of motion around a joint, it has more space to absorb and distribute incoming forces around the knee area. Many of the knee injuries that we discuss are a direct result of tight, non-flexible muscles that don't give your knee any space to move.

Multiple muscles pass all around the knee joint. Whether your calf, thigh, hamstrings, quadriceps, gastrocnemius, or soleus, they all work together to flex, extend, and stabilize the knee. If some muscles are tight and inflexible, the exact source of pain won't be always obvious. This is why you might want to think about stretching the tissues around the knees, making yourself supple and loose.

I discuss the best stretching exercises for the knee in depth later, but one last point that I'd like to make to those who are still on the fence about stretching is that becoming more flexible actually makes you stronger. That might sound odd at first, but think about it: you can only strengthen with the flexibility that you have. When a muscle contracts, the two sides of the muscle fiber come together to produce a force, which is your power. If the muscles are very close together, you produce a certain amount of power, but if you stretch your muscles so that the muscle fibers are wider apart, they will produce more force, or power, when they come together. For example, if you produce a contraction from your tight quads by extending your knee, you might produce a power of, for example, ten. But if your muscles were more supple and flexible, there would be more muscle available to produce power with the same knee extension, this time producing twenty instead of ten. Improving your flexibility will help decrease your knee pain.

## MUSCLE IMBALANCES

Muscle imbalances are big contributors to all sorts of knee problems, and we hear this term used quite frequently. But what does it really mean? Simply put, muscle imbalances occur when one muscle is stronger than its opposing muscle, normally located on the opposite side of the stronger muscle. Imbalance in strength and flexibility might be between your legs, with one leg being stronger or more dominant than the other, or perhaps your quads are stronger than your hamstrings on one leg. Another major imbalance that many runners, cyclists, and others experience is strong muscles on the outer, or lateral, part of their leg muscle, like the vastus lateralis of the quads and the IT band versus the weak or underused inner part of their legs, which consist of the vastus medialis of the quads and the adductor muscles. This is a common problem that occurs when you play the same sport all the time and those muscles develop really well, while the other muscles are not developed at all. All muscles need to be developed because the human body needs to be in balance or problems will arise. There can be other types of imbalances that can occur; for example, placing weight on one leg to compensate for an injury on the other leg. If you don't correct the injured leg quickly, you'll start to feel discomfort in your back due to changes in gait or walking patterns, and things can only get worse. Seeing a doctor, physical therapist, or allied health professional sooner rather than later is the best gift that you can give yourself.

## PREVIOUS INJURIES

Old injuries can be a recurrent issue. You might have experienced a knee injury a while ago, did some stuff for it, thinking the pain went away for a while, but, all of a sudden, it comes back with a vengeance. Why does the pain come back? My question would then be, was the problem that caused the pain ever resolved in the first place? Some of the reasons that prior injuries could impact healing may be

1. incomplete rehab: Maybe your leg musculature is not as strong or flexible as it needs to be.
2. strenuous activity done too soon: We are all victims of this, myself included. We all want to return to our favorite sport or activity, even if we are not ready physically to perform at that level.
3. improper warm up: This almost falls into item 2 above. You might think that you do not need to warm up, but that's when injuries can start.
4. not eating well: Nutrition is important in giving you the energy you need to perform at your best.
5. overtraining: I have many patients who believe that training seven days a week or doing their exercises three or four times a day will make them better, stronger, and heal faster. They forget that healing and getting the strength you need also comes from proper rest and sleep and not pushing yourself too hard.

*Chapter 2*

## POOR CONDITIONING

Your conditioning is very important to the health of your knee and other joints. If you are out of shape or not in adequate physical and aerobic shape, then eventually your body and joints start to break down. One of the ways that you might be in poor condition is that your legs and torso are not very strong and stable. If that is the case, there is a very strong possibility that if you do any movement in everyday life, especially if you are not used to doing that movement, an injury may occur. Most of us have desk jobs where we sit all day without moving much, and over time, our muscles become loose and weak. Imagine if that's compounded by sitting on the couch watching TV at night after work. After a while, simply getting up from the couch or walking to the corner store becomes a bigger effort than before, and problems can arise from it. Your back and knees stiffen up, leading you to not want to move again. I call this the "couch potato syndrome."

I believe that you start working out in a slow and consistent manner. Come September or January, too many people want to get into shape quickly, push themselves harder than they should, and work out

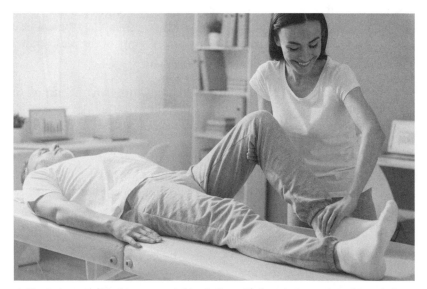

A Physiotherapist Working on an Athlete's Knee. *Zinkevych, image from Bigstockphoto. com*

intensely every day. This is asking for trouble because the body doesn't have a chance to rest and grow. Working our bodies aerobically is also something that we should do, because muscles need oxygen to grow and perform, and a strong blood flow takes nourishment to all the parts of the body. If the body isn't nourished, it becomes weak, which therefore increases the risk of injury.

## WHAT IS TENDONITIS?

Before we understand what tendonitis is, we need to know the definition of *-itis*. A suffix derived from the Greek language, *-itis* means inflammation of a structure. For example, tendonitis is an inflammation of a tendon. The inflammation is caused when the tendon is pulled or stretched past what it can absorb. That is what tendonitis—as well as "sprain" and "strain"—really means: the structure has been overstretched to the point of injury.

Capsulitis is inflammation of a capsule due to excessive rubbing of the capsule and tendon, muscles, or ligaments that should not be rubbing that way. An example is a patellofemoral joint in plica syndrome, which we discuss later in this chapter.

Bursitis is the inflammation of your bursa, saclike structures cushioning, absorbing pressure, and helping two structures or surfaces to "glide," normally a muscle and a bone. The knee has eleven bursa found all around the knee. Again, due to excessive rubbing from tendons or muscles, bursa can become inflamed and swollen.

## WHAT IS PAIN?

What is pain, really? It is described as a highly unpleasant physical sensation caused by illness or injury. Because describing how we perceive pain and our tolerance for pain differs from one person to another, it is difficult to describe and define properly. Pain is a signal or sensation that comes from your nerves. Keeping in mind that pain is a signal to the brain that something is wrong, it is important to figure out what is causing the pain, rather than simply treating it. After a doctor has ruled out non-musculoskeletal problems (e.g., fractures, dislocations, or other medical conditions), and your pain has been classified as tendonitis, it is up to your therapist to look at two major things: (1) how is the range of motion (ROM) of your knee and all the structures around it, and (2) how is your knee's overall strength (i.e., are there imbalances of strength and flexibility that should be addressed?). When someone has a properly medically diagnosed knee problem, merely taking medication or doing a random exercise routine will not fix the ailment. A combined approach of reducing the inflammation with medication if necessary or by icing the area, along with ROM and strength exercises and a good proprioception routine, will improve your overall condition and reduce pain.

What is most important to me when seeing patients is knowing the deficiencies in their knee's range of motion and where their lack of strength or imbalance around the knee is. This is the information I try to get when I see a patient for the first time during their initial evaluation. What's tight, weak, and strong in the area or what isn't working the way it should be is my primary focus when I examine my patient. I work on those things first before looking at anything else.


## WHAT CAUSES TENDONITIS?

Tendonitis is usually caused by minor, repetitive, incorrect movements done frequently each day. Anyone can get tendonitis, but it is most common between the ages of twenty to forty, and it occurs when the tendon has been pulled more than it is accustomed to.

The amount of wear and tear on the tendons is generally higher among individuals involved in athletics, specifically sports such as rugby, football, or rowing. The tendons of the knee often become inflamed due to overuse of the knee or trauma involving the knee joint. Such knee injuries are commonly noted in individuals who are involved in different kinds of sports.

### Tendinitis versus Tendinosis

*Tendinitis* and *tendinosis* are two terms that you might have heard before but don't really know the difference between them. Let's start with the ends of the words: *-itis* means inflammation (redness, swelling, heat, soreness, and achiness) of a particular tendon, like patellar tendinitis; however, *-osis* refers to a chronic degeneration without any inflammation. Tendinitis is the inflammation of the tendon and results

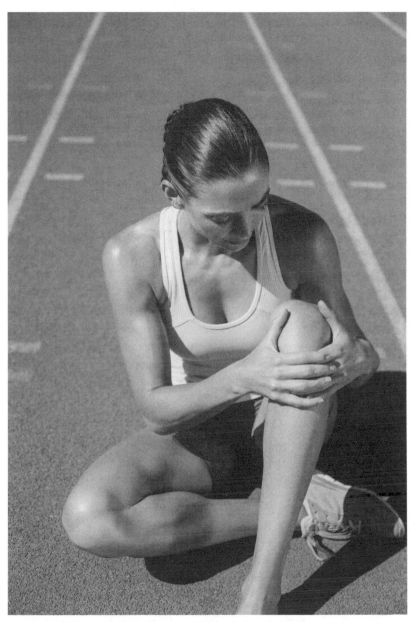

Female Athlete with Pain. *Wavebreak Media Ltd., image from Bigstockphoto.com*

from micro-tears that occur when the musculotendinous unit is over-loaded with a force that is too great and/or too sudden. It is usually due to continual, repetitive movements. Tendinitis happens in the acute stage, whereas tendinosis happens at the chronic stage.

Tendinosis is a degeneration of the tendon's collagen fibers in response to chronic overuse. It can be called chronic tendinitis. When tendons are overused without allowing any time to rest and heal, which happens often with repetitive strain types of injuries, tendinosis occurs. Even small movements that you wouldn't think are a big deal, like clicking your computer's mouse, can cause tendinosis,when done repeatedly.

The healing time for tendinitis is several days to six weeks, depending on when treatment started.

Let's cover some of the common knee injuries that affect so many people.

## PATELLAR TENDONITIS (JUMPER'S KNEE)

Patellar tendonitis, also called jumper's knee, is one of the most common knee injuries out there. It is an overuse injury that can cause inflammation or irritation of the patellar tendon, which is located below your kneecap. It is one of the largest and strongest tendons of the body. It is called jumper's knee because it frequently occurs during jumping and landing activities and sports such as basketball and volleyball. When you jump, the quadriceps muscles give an explosive force of contraction, which straightens the knee and pushes you up into the air. When you are coming down to land, your quadriceps muscles absorb the landing forces by allowing a small amount of controlled eccentric knee bend. Repetitive jumping or landing starts to put pressure and strain on the patella tendon. At first, the strain might be minimal and not cause many issues. What happens is that while you continue practicing your sport and ignoring the pain, you may continue to strain the tendon. The patellar tendon starts to overstretch and the damage progressively becomes worse, causing pain and dysfunction. Patellar tendonitis is the result of your tendon not being strong enough for the demands and pressures of your sport or activity.

Some of the complaints that people who have this problem experience are pain on the front, side, or, in most cases, below the kneecap near the bone that the patellar tendon attaches itself to. The pain might feel like a dull ache in the beginning but might become more sensitive as the micro-tears increase due to small pulls on the tendon. You initially might start to feel it after a basketball or volleyball game, but when as it worsens, you might feel it continually throughout the day. In my experience, the cause can be tight muscles that don't give the patella enough space to move or perhaps the entire knee area is tight and not flexible. If every muscle is pulling tightly on the knee, there isn't much space or wiggle room to allow for movement.

Another major issue is muscle imbalance. If some muscles are stronger than others, then they pull the patella one way, but the other, weaker muscles won't be able to pull it back to the middle, which can also cause the tendinitis. If this continues for a couple of weeks or longer, the tendinitis is now considered tendinopathy, which takes longer to heal and return to normal.

So what can you do to help yourself? I believe in a good stretching program involving the quads, hamstring, and calf muscles, as well as some eccentric exercises to build up strength and provide stability and security when coming down from a basketball layup or a volleyball spike. It is also a good idea to see a physical therapist or allied health professional to help you with pain relief and get you back into your sport.

## PATELLOFEMORAL PAIN SYNDROME (PFPS)

Patellofemoral pain syndrome (PFPS) is sometimes known as runner's knee or chondromalacia, where underneath or the back part of the kneecap rubs against the side of the cartilage of the femur, causing pain and irritation. This is the situation in which you can hear your knees cracking and popping when you are going up and down the stairs, squatting, or getting up from sitting on the floor. Likewise, you can hear someone else who has it from across the hall.

Some of the major factors associated with this condition include muscular imbalances of the quadriceps, weak glutes, and tight muscles around the knee.

### Muscular Imbalances of the Quadriceps

If your vastus lateralis and iliotibial (IT) band are strong but also very tight, and the vastus medialis and adductor muscles are loose and weak, when you contract your quads, your vastus lateralis contracts before your medialis, which pulls your patella out of alignment with the patellar groove found on your femur. Why are your outside muscles stronger than your inside muscles? I believe that, to some extent, we are built this way. When we walk or run, our leg moves forward, then outside, back, and forward again. It doesn't need that much strength or power to come toward the middle of the body. Think of ice skating or roller blading, when the leg pushes hard to go to the outside but not as hard to come to the inside. I believe that this might be one of the reasons for the imbalance.

## Weak Glutes

When I was a student therapist, I thought that if you treated the knee joint, a knee injury would get better. Sometimes, that worked, but most times it did not. I couldn't figure out why. Now, I know that if you have weak glute muscles, more often than not, you will also have some knee pain.

There are three gluteus or butt muscles: the gluteus maximus, the one most people know about; the gluteus medius; and the gluteus minimus. Although all three muscles are weak, I focus primarily on the gluteus medius muscle here.

So why would a weak gluteus medius muscle contribute to knee pain? Most of the things that we do in life, whether walking, running, or even going up and down stairs, we do on one leg. Let's talk first about the leg that you are standing on or the one supporting your weight when you move. The gluteus medius, on the leg that is supporting your weight, pulls that side of your pelvis down toward the floor to keep the unsupported side of the pelvis up. If the gluteus medius muscle is weak on the standing leg, your pelvis will experience more banging and jarring sensations with every step. If your pelvis isn't stabilized in a neutral position when standing on that leg, something gives way eventually. On the downside leg, the gluteus medius also pulls the thigh (and effectively the knee) outward to prevent the leg from collapsing toward the other leg. This is extremely important for balancing all the different forces throughout your knee and for maintaining proper tracking of the kneecap or patella. When your knee falls inward or adducts like that, it can put a lot of pressure and strain on your medial collateral ligament (MCL), which causes the development of inner knee pain. It can also change the way you walk, which is called Trendelenburg gait. By preventing the knees from collapsing inward, your gluteus medius and gluteus maximus can reduce ACL-related sprains, because when your knee falls inward, it also puts a lot of pressure on your ACL. It is important to strengthen your glutes because they help keep your pelvis in a neutral position and reduce unnecessary stress on your joints.

How do our glutes get so weak to begin with? One of the reasons why the glutes get weak is likely due to the nature of our work. More and more people have desk jobs in front of a computer, and we sit all day. We squish our tush all day, and we don't really use it. When you don't use it, you lose it. So, we lose strength in our glutes and hamstring muscles, and they become weak and inactive. We also have a tendency to lean forward, therefore tightening our hip flexors and quads, which stretches the glutes and hamstrings. Stretching out our hip flexors and quads as well as strengthening our glutes and hamstrings provides better balance in our bodies, and our knees will thank us.

A knee that falls inward will also change the position of your ankle, making you more flatfooted or pronated than you should be. It has been shown through research that a weak gluteus medius is related to ankle sprains, so working and strengthening your gluteus medius muscle can help stabilize your ankles and reduce ankle injuries by not allowing your body to move too far outward past the ankle. It's about balance, not just strength.

## Tight Muscles around the Knee

No one likes to stretch. It isn't fun. People don't think it is needed, but that is far from the truth. Stretching decreases pressure on and around the knee. It gives you more space to move and balances you out. For example, a tight quadriceps muscle puts a lot of pressure on the patella by pulling it upward and not allowing it to come down when you flex your knee, causing pain and discomfort. Tight hamstrings can place force through the back part of the knee, pushing the femur bone into the patella and increasing pressure between the two bones, which creates less space to move. A tight calf muscle causes the back part of your foot to pronate too much. As the leg moves over the foot at the ankle, the ankle reaches its end range of motion early and will not go any further if the calf muscle is tight. The only way the leg can go further is if the midfoot (arch) collapses. This can only happen if the back part of the foot pronates even more, causing overpronation, leading to ankle sprain, as well as making your knee go inward in a valgus position, instead of a midline position.

IT band tightness also can cause PFPS. The IT band, located on the outside part of the leg, can put a lot of pressure or force on the outside part of the patella and externally rotate the tibia, which can upset the balance of the patellofemoral mechanism. A tight IT band and weak adductor and vastus medialis muscles pull the kneecap to the outside, rather than staying in the patellar groove on the femur where the patella is supposed to pass through.

## OSGOOD-SCHLATTER DISEASE (OSD)

Osgood-Schlatter disease (OSD) is not really a disease, but a common cause of knee pain in growing children. It occurs in boys around the ages of thirteen or fourteen and in girls at ages eleven or twelve. It is more common in boys, but as more girls become involved in sports, it is also seen in them. OSD is an inflammation or irritation of the area just below the knee, where the patellar tendon attaches to the tibia. This area is called a tibial tuberosity, and it becomes a bump that is sore to the touch and swollen. When the tuberosity gets overloaded through exercise like squats, jumping, or running, it starts to split apart a bit. When the muscle fibers try to connect and heal, the area gets thicker and eventually forms scar tissue. This happens to certain adolescents who are going through a growth spurt while playing sports on an everyday basis.

OSD most often occurs during growth spurts, when bones, muscles, tendons, and other structures are changing rapidly. Because physical activity puts additional stress on bones and muscles, children who participate in athletics—especially running and jumping sports—are at increased risk for this condition. However, less active adolescents may also experience OSD. The problem normally decreases and vanishes completely once the child has stopped growing.

A physical therapist or other allied health professional can show your child how to stretch the quadriceps and hamstring muscles, which reduces the strain and pulling where the kneecap's tendon attaches to the tibial tuberosity. Also, performing some specific strengthening exercises for the quadriceps muscle can help increase stability of the knee. Resting as well as icing the knee also can help with the pain.

## MENISCAL TEARS

The menisci are the shock absorbers of the knee. They cushion the tibia when pressure is applied from the femur or vice versa; for example, when we climb up and down stairs, jump, run, or do anything else that allows bones to come in contact with each other. Meniscus tears are a special risk for older athletes, since the meniscus weakens with age. It is estimated that more than 40 percent of people ages sixty-five or older have meniscal tears. The outer third of the meniscus, often referred to as the "red zone," has a good blood flow and can sometimes even heal on its own if the tear is small. However, the inner two thirds of the meniscus, known as the "white zone," does not have a good blood supply.

When we talk about a meniscal injury, we normally talk about meniscal tears. Tears happen due to trauma, degeneration, or overuse. Of the two menisci, it is often the medial meniscus that gets injured more than the lateral meniscus. This is due to anatomy. The medial meniscus is on the wall of the knee capsule, so when a force comes at it, the medial meniscus takes a direct hit. It is also connected to the MCL ligament. The lateral meniscus is not, nor is it connected to the lateral collateral ligament (LCL), so it has more room to maneuver.

A meniscal tear may be in the anterior horn, body, or posterior horn of the meniscus. A posterior horn tear is one we see the most in our clinic. There are different shapes of meniscal tears. The way that the meniscal shape is formed lets the doctor and therapist know how to treat it. Some of the most common types of tears follow.

A bucket handle or longitudinal tear is a tear that is almost a straight line down the inner rim of the meniscus. Try picturing a handle on a bucket. You can flip that handle from side to side. The same type of thing also happens inside your knee. The entire meniscus tears, and the C-shaped disc flips over and sits in front of the knee. These tears usually occur in areas with good blood supply to the meniscus. When treated early (within three weeks), such tears generally can be repaired fully. It is possible that the meniscus can be displaced, but surgery for that can successfully repair it. The cartilage that makes up the menisci weakens the older you get, making the menisci prone to degeneration and tearing. Older individuals can get a meniscal tear as result of a minor injury, such as doing a quick movement while walking and missing a step, or from the up-and-down motion of walking stairs. Such tears are not something that you did wrong; these tears are commonly part of the overall condition of osteoarthritis of the knee as you grow older. When the menisci start to degenerate, they become torn in every direction.

A parrot beak or radial tear is a tear that forms when the meniscus splits in two directions due to repetitive stress activities such as running. This oblique type of tear is often called a parrot beak tear, since it resembles a parrot's beak. Oblique tears are a combination of both radial and longitudinal tears, in that they lie perpendicular to the edge of the meniscus but then curve in such a way that a portion lies parallel to the C-shaped fibers of the meniscus.

A meniscal tear is usually classified as "complete" or "incomplete." A tear is considered complete if it goes all the way through the meniscus, separating a piece of the tissue from the rest of the meniscus. If the tear is still partly attached to the body of the meniscus, it is considered incomplete. Tears are also classified as either "stable" or "unstable." A stable tear does not move and may heal on its own. An unstable tear allows the meniscus to move abnormally and is likely to become a problem if not surgically corrected.

### How Do I Know if I Injured My Meniscus?

While doing a sport or activity, you might hear a "pop" or "click" and feel pain on the inside of your knee between your tibia and femur, called the medial joint line. You may also get pain in the back and outside of the knee, referred to as posterior lateral knee pain.

The pain and discomfort that you experience may be a sharp, stabbing sensation rather than a constant dull ache. You would feel it more intensely when bending the knee deeply or fully straightening your leg. Twisting your body on the knee with your foot planted on the floor may also hurt. If you find that you have difficulty straightening your knee, it could mean that you have a torn meniscus, and going to your doctor right away might be a very smart thing to do. If you hear clicking in your knee, it is not the same as "locking," and surgery is probably not needed. Unless the doctor absolutely says that you need surgery, it is best to try the conservative route with your physiotherapist to work on the swelling, pain, and even locking with therapy sessions. It might take seven to ten days for a minor meniscal injury or up to two or three months to fully recover from a major meniscal tear, but I believe that is better than going the surgical route.

## LIGAMENT INJURIES

The purpose of your ligaments is to connect and keep together the bones of your knee, connecting your femur to your lower bones firmly and not giving any abnormal laxity, sway, or instability. Ligaments are made of tough bands of tissue, but if enough outside force is placed on them, they can be pulled or stretched. When the ligament is pulled, it is called a sprain. There are typically three grades to determine the level of a knee sprain.

Grade 1 sprains are usually mild or light sprains in which only 10 percent of the fibers actually are damaged. Although the fibers might have been stretched, the rest are doing fine and can still keep your knee stable. During a clinical exam, you won't find that the knee is loose when the doctor or therapist performs some laxity tests.

Grade 2 sprains comprise the bulk of the sprains that therapists see, wherein the patient is in obvious pain and has difficulty walking properly with a normal walk. With a grade 2 sprain, anywhere from 10 to 90 percent of the fibers may be damaged and stretched out, but the ligament is still connected to both sides of the bone. Your doctor might classify it as a partial ligament tear.

There is both good and bad news regarding grade 3 sprains. The good news is that you probably won't feel as much pain as you would with a grade 2 sprain, but I would not wish for such a sprain. A grade 3 sprain means that the ligament is completely torn apart, split into two separate pieces. This is called a complete ligament tear. With such a sprain, you would definitely have significant instability in your knee and you would not want to walk around. Depending on whether there is additional shredding of the ligament, surgery is probably required with this level of injury.

When one of your knee ligaments gets a serious sprain, there is a possibility that other parts of the knee may also be injured due to its anatomy. Some ligaments and structures are connected to each other. For example, because the MCL helps to protect the ACL from all the forces acting on your knee, the ACL can get pulled when the MCL is torn. In more than half the cases of a grade 2 or 3 MCL sprain diagnosis, the ACL also is sprained.

Let's look at these ligament injuries more closely.

### Collateral Ligaments

You have two collateral ligaments on the sides of your knee: the MCL, or medial collateral ligament, and the LCL, or lateral collateral ligament.

*Medial Collateral Ligament*

This is a ligament that is located on the inside part of your knee, and it connects the femur bone to the tibia. The MCL has both superficial and deep attachments. The superficial MCL fibers attach proximally to the femur and distally to the inside part of the tibia, approximately four centimeters below the knee joint line. The deep MCL fibers start from the medial joint capsule and are attached to the medial meniscus. Its job or function is to prevent the knee from bending inward. If there is a direct blow to the outside of your knee that is more than what your MCL can absorb, you will get a sprained or pulled ligament.

With a grade 1 sprain of your MCL, you will feel pain when the site of the damage is touched. If you push on the ligament when the knee is slightly bent and the shin is moved inward in relation to the thigh, it will cause pain and discomfort.

With a grade 2 sprain, the pain will be worse when the area is touched and when the ligament is placed under stress. The knee joint usually swells, but it might take up to twenty-four hours for that to show up.

If you are unlucky enough to get a grade 3 sprain, in which your ligament is completely torn apart, the knee joint will be unstable and you cannot continue your activity. You will probably see some bruising and some accumulation of fluid in the joint. However, because the knee capsule that surrounds the joint is also damaged, this fluid may leak out and swelling may not be evident right away. Even though most of these types of injuries are treated with surgery, now some of them are treated nonoperatively, especially if only the MCL is injured and the ACL and medial meniscus are fine. If two or more structures are torn, then surgery is done. In the past, a nonoperative treatment for such an injury would have been a long leg cast. Now, standard practice is to brace the knee with a hinged or bent-knee orthosis. Some medical surgeons prefer waiting up to six weeks with the knee at 30 degrees of flexion, which is the knee's resting position, before starting therapy, but protocols vary depending on the surgeon. Crutches are usually necessary for one or two weeks.

*What Should You Do When You Have an MCL Injury?*

The most important things that you should do is reducing the pain and stabilizing your knee. Some of the actions that you should do include:

- applying ice to reduce swelling and pain;
- elevating your knee above your heart to help reduce swelling;
- taking nonsteroidal anti-inflammatory drugs (NSAIDs) to ease pain and swelling, as prescribed by your doctor;
- compressing your knee using an elastic bandage or brace, which keeps everything together and prevents your knee from ballooning out;
- resting your leg—please do it;
- using crutches to keep weight off your injured knee.

After that, it would be wise to seek out your physical therapist, who can help you with a proper rehabilitation plan.

### The Million Dollar Question: How Long Does It Take to Heal an MCL Injury?

Your recovery time depends on the severity of your MCL injury. Since grade 1 MCL injuries are not that bad, they only take from seven to ten days to fully heal. Grade 2 injuries, however, can take much longer to heal —up to four or five weeks (so don't get upset at your therapist!). Grade 3 injuries are the most severe and have the longest recovery time. It typically takes eight to ten weeks or more for these types of injuries to heal.

### Lateral Collateral Ligament

The lateral collateral ligament, or LCL, is a thin band of cartilage located on the outside part of your knee. It starts on the femur and ends at the top part of the fibula bone. Its purpose is to brace and stop your knee from a varus force, which is a force pushing the knee from the medial or inner side of the knee area, causing stress to the outside of the knee. An example of this would be a direct blow to the inside of the knee or the knee being pushed away from the body with the foot planted. The good news is that this ligament is more flexible than the MCL because it connects neither to the capsule of the knee nor the lateral meniscus, as the MCL does.

Symptoms of an LCL sprain are localized pain on the outside part of the knee, difficulty walking, swelling, and discomfort. If the impact to the LCL is great enough, it also can cause damage to the peroneal nerve, which causes your foot to drop, making it difficult to bring your foot toward you.

The protocol for treating the LCL is the same as treating the MCL. Physical therapists concentrate mostly on reducing pain, restoring the full range of motion (ROM) in your knee, as well as strengthening the muscles in the area to regain your lost stability.

## Cruciate Ligaments

There are two ligaments that cross between the back part of the knee and the front. They are the posterior cruciate ligament (PCL) and the anterior cruciate ligament (ACL).

### Posterior Cruciate Ligament

This ligament is located at the back of the knee. It connects the front part of the femur to the back part of the tibia (*cruciate* means "cross"). Its main purpose is to stop the tibia from moving backward on the femur. Between the ACL and PCL is the knee capsule, and a synovial membrane covers them both individually.

The most common way of injuring your PCL is by a direct blow to a bent knee, such as hitting the knee on the dashboard in a car accident or falling down hard on your knee, which forces your tibia backward on your femur. Although a blow to your posterior cruciate ligament will probably cause less pain, disability, and knee instability than an ACL tear, it can still sideline you for several weeks or months. Some of the related symptoms include pain and discomfort. Your knee might swell up significantly within hours of your injury, but the most significant symptom might be the feeling that your leg is giving out or giving way. It is entirely possible that you are fine at the time of injury, but as the day progresses, your condition worsens. Please see your doctor as soon as possible or go to the hospital where trained staff can evaluate you properly. One of the reasons for this is because you might have experienced another knee injury along with the PCL problem. These include cartilage/meniscus injuries, bone bruises, ACL tears, fractures, posterolateral injuries, and collateral ligament injuries.

Due to the PCL's strength, only a violent force causes the area to stretch or tear. The most common cause is a motor vehicle accident in which your knee slams into the car's dashboard. The force would hit your bent knee, pushing your tibia violently backward against your femur and therefore causing your PCL to tear. Seatbelts can help prevent knee injuries, too. PCL injuries can also happen in sports, specifically football and soccer, where players may fall down on a bent knee while their ankle is pointed downward. The tibia slams into the ground first and moves backward. Being tackled when your knee is bent can also cause this injury.

As with ligament sprains, there are also three grades of PCL tears.

A grade 1 tear is a tear in which a small number of fibers in the PCL are stretched, creating microscopic tears in the ligament. This injury is considered minor and does not significantly affect the knee's ability to support your weight.

A grade 2 tear is a more severe and painful injury, wherein the PCL is partially torn and the knee is relatively unstable, which means it gives out periodically when standing or walking. Some of the fibers are still intact, while some are completely torn.

With a grade 3 tear, the PCL is either completely torn apart or separated at its end from the bone that it normally connects to, making the knee completely unstable and placing significant strain on the other ligaments around it. As mentioned earlier, it usually takes a great deal of force to cause a severe PCL injury; patients with grade 3 PCL sprains often also tear their ACL, menisci, or collateral ligaments as well. Extensive therapy is needed to return the patient to full sporting activity, and surgery may be required to reattach the ligament to the bone, as well as to repair any other structures that might be involved.

The recovery time for a PCL injury depends on the severity of the injury, as well as whether any other structures are involved, but a full recovery can take from four months up to a full year.

### Anterior Cruciate Ligament

This is probably the most talked about ligament in the knee, with countless rehabilitation protocols for and research about it.

The ACL connects the back part of the femur to the front part of the tibia. A small part of the ACL connects to the medial meniscus and MCL. Its main function is to prevent anterior, or forward movement, of the tibia off the femur, as well as to prevent your leg from hyperextending, or bending backward instead of forward. The ACL also helps protect the knee from excessive valgus pressure, which is when the knee bends inward toward the body, such as when a football player is tackled from the side. The ACL also provides roughly 90 percent the knee joint's stability. When the ACL is stretched or torn, the knee can feel very unstable and can oftentimes "give way," swell, and become painful. An ACL tear can be part of a knee injury that is referred to as "the terrible triad," which also includes tearing of the MCL and medial meniscus. ACL tears are graded the same as PCL tears, which are described in the PCL section.

Most ACL tears are a result of landing or planting in cutting or pivoting sports, as in basketball or football, with or without contact. Most serious athletes require an ACL surgical reconstruction if they have a complete tear and want to return to sports because the ACL is crucial for stabilizing the knee when turning or planting. Depending on the severity of the tear and how the ligament was injured, the recovery time can be one to two years or longer.

The ACL can be treated nonoperatively with strengthening, ROM exercises, and specific physical therapy if it is not completely torn and the knee is still stable or if the patient is not participating in any sports or activities that use cutting and pivoting movements.

The most important part of any ACL nonoperative treatment is strengthening the muscles around the knee, especially the hamstrings. Physical therapy is vital to any ACL surgery. Completely recovering and getting ready to return to competitive sports or other activities typically takes about six to nine months, depending on the surgery.

The early stages of rehab therapy, which lasts approximately six weeks, primarily focuses on getting and maintaining full knee ROM as well as preventing scar tissue. The second part of rehab is directed toward regaining knee strength in every direction until the patient feels comfortable performing activities of daily living, like walking, jogging, and bending without fear. Finally, sports-specific rehabilitation is provided to athletes or weekend warriors returning to their sport.

If the doctor recommends ACL surgery, he or she may prescribe "prehab" before operating, since many studies show that acquiring good range of motion and increasing muscular strength and stability of the knee only helps the patient to get better faster and with less physiotherapy needed after the surgery.

ACL reconstruction surgery has a 90 percent success rate in terms of stability of your knee and the full return to your sport or activity. ACL reconstruction surgery also seems to help protect the menisci from future injury, as well as to slow degenerative changes in the knee joint in the years ahead. ACL surgical reconstruction is very expensive: surgery, the surgeon and anesthesiologist's fees, and physical therapy can cost $10,000 to $15,000.

Women are four to six times more likely to get ACL injuries than men playing the same sport at the same level. There are a few reasons for this. Women tend to have an imbalance in the strength ratio between their quadriceps and hamstring muscles. Female athletes are more likely to use their quadriceps muscle to slow down from a sprint rather than their glutes and hamstrings, which causes an instability in the knee joint. Male athletes are more likely to slow down using their hamstrings. This slight difference provides significant protection to the ligaments of the knee.

I believe that women who play soccer, basketball, or any other high-level sport should warm up differently from men. Training their hamstrings and glutes before playing, as well as running backward instead of forward, could greatly help female athletes avoid knee problems. Ground-level programs for women have started, and hopefully, this becomes the everyday way of thinking for coaches and athletes alike.

## SUMMARY

- There are different risk factors pertaining to knee problems: age, gender, muscle imbalances, weight, and poor conditioning.
- Muscle imbalances are a major contributor to most knee issues. The muscles located on the outside of the knee are stronger than the ones located on the inside, causing the patella to shift to the outside. This misalignment may be one of the reasons for the cracking or popping of the patella on the groove of the femur.
- Strengthening the glute muscles, specifically the gluteus medius, plays a significant role in the treatment of patellofemoral pain syndrome. When the gluteus medius is strengthened, it prohibits the knee from dropping inward, keeping the leg straight.
- Women are built differently than men. Aside from their larger Q angle due to their wider hips, their quads are much stronger than their hamstrings, unlike men. This imbalance causes more knee injuries, specifically ACL injuries. Recommendations suggest that training should concentrate on the hamstrings and glutes rather than the quadriceps. Also, when warming up, female athletes should practice running backward to better contract the hamstring and glute muscles and to stretch out the quad muscles. This will reduce the number of knee injuries.

# 3

# My Knee Is Shot!

The aim of the wise is not to secure pleasure, but to avoid pain.

—Aristotle

Gymnastics is Kayla's world. From the moment she stepped onto the floor mat and learned how to tumble as a young girl, she was hooked. She balances on the high beam, jumps off the springboard with ease, and does cartwheels and somersaults as if she was born to do so. She was a natural and thought that she can do gymnastics forever. But at a qualifications event, she missed her footing on the balance beam and landed awkwardly on the floor with her leg buckling inward as she landed. She immediately felt a stabbing pain go through her body, and she could barely move. When the doctor told her that the sharp pain was due to an MCL sprain and she would be out of the competition, she thought her life was over.

We all love doing our own thing. Whether we are jumping up to score a basket, running in a marathon, or bending down to tend to the flowers in the garden, we use our knees a lot. Run, jump, twist, stop, and start—our knees take the brunt of all that pressure. Research has shown that more than 100 million Americans suffer from chronic knee and joint pain, making knee pain the second most common cause of chronic pain, after lower back and neck pain.

There are two types of knee pain: traumatic and nontraumatic. Traumatic knee injuries can result from a violent collision, like a car accident, or from a fall from a great height, in which the damage, like fractures or dislocations, is obvious to find and diagnose. They can also happen in sports; for example, when a football player tackles another player, pushing his knee toward the inside, called a chop block. Traumatic injuries can

37

also occur when landing awkwardly, twisting your knee as you land, after a basketball layup. A traumatic knee injury is really any force applied to the knee that is greater than what the knee can absorb.

Far less obvious are nontraumatic injuries to the knee region. One day, the knee feels a little stiff and sore after playing a game of hockey with the boys. You might rub the spot in pain a bit and return to what you were doing, confident that it will go away. A couple of days later, the discomfort is back. It's even worse, and you can barely walk. You bend the knee and try to get the kinks out, and it feels a little better. Back to what you were doing. Ouch! It still hurts. Your movements are constrained, limited. But what can you do? You have no idea how it happened. You didn't fall, didn't plow into something, nothing collided with you. Yet the pain, when it happens, is hot and sharp. Each time it strikes, it startles you with its intensity.

This is the kind of pain that builds over time—just as the initial injury to your knee undoubtedly happened, little by little, over time. How did it happen? Most likely through bad posture and body mechanics. Look at the position of your body or the way you carry yourself when standing or sitting. Do you have a desk job or work at a computer, all day? Does your job consist of lifting hefty objects or going up and down flights of stairs every day? Do you play sports frequently and don't really have the time or desire to stretch afterward? You already have bad muscle imbalances and ignore the pain: "Suck it up and play through the pain," your friends say. Over time, these eventualities can end up affecting the knee joint and causing those sudden, dramatic bursts of knee pain.

Since you can't recall a reason for the pain, you think it will go away by itself. The bad news is that it won't—as you well know by now, which is why you're reading this book.

So how can you deal with the agony and get yourself on the road to fixing your knee quickly, confidently, and effectively?

## PAIN IS A SIGNAL

The very first thing to do is to acknowledge the pain and accept it for what it is—a signal that your body is trying to tell you that something is wrong with your knee. You probably have felt that pain and would have no trouble recognizing the signal; you *know* something is horribly wrong.

Pain is one of the body's best ways to communicate between the brain and the injured area. It is the body's way of protecting itself from causing real harm. Pain acts as a warning signal that tissues are being damaged, which forces you to remove yourself from the source of pain. What would happen to our fingers if we couldn't feel pain when placing our hands on a hot stove or touching a sharp object? We definitely would have suffered unnecessary damage to ourselves. The purpose of pain is really to protect you, not to hurt you. Think of it as your body's internal alarm system.

On the other hand, pain can create severe discomfort and unpleasant sensory and emotional feelings. Every person experiences pain differently; some are able to handle the feeling whereas others are totally incapacitated by it.

The two major categories of pain can be classified as *acute* and *chronic*. According to Segen's medical dictionary, acute pain is described as "a normal, physiological and usually time-limited response to adverse (noxious) chemical, thermal or mechanical stimulus."[1] Acute pain normally happens immediately after an injury and lasts for twenty-four to forty-eight hours. It is usually created by a particular injury or physical ailment that can be treated—once we figure out where the problem is.

Acute physical pain can result from a sprain in your knee, from a quick movement, or from lifting something that's too heavy. Making a wrong move can cause acute pain to shoot through a specific area of your body, like your knee. There are many ways of experiencing acute pain, from stubbing your foot in a door to having a major accident.

Subacute pain is a bit harder to define. It is somewhere between acute and chronic pain, and it is more common than people realize. We often see people in subacute pain in the clinic.

Subacute pain normally begins forty-eight to seventy-two hours after the initial injury and can last, if not properly treated, for months. At this stage, after the inflammation part has occurred during the initial acute phase, the body starts to do the repair work on the injured area. Work on the "construction site" begins by laying down some new tissue in the form of collagen. In the beginning, this collagen is very "immature" and a little disorganized. It takes, on average, six to eight weeks to fully mature the region. The way we decide that an area has healed is when it reaches a level at which it can handle the load that it did before the injury, when it regains its full range of motion, and when there is no longer any pain in that area.

Chronic pain begins at approximately six months or so after an injury. Studies have shown that those who suffer chronic pain experience changes in their personality, with sharper than normal mood swings, increased depression, as well as feelings ranging from anxiety to suicidal tendencies. Stress and pain can become a vicious cycle that can be hard to escape. When you are in pain, you feel more stressed and anxious. The anxiety and stress can cause your muscles to tense up, which increases the pain even more. Therefore, it is always better to see a health specialist sooner rather than later, and the idea that "it will go away on its own" is not something to rely on.

Pain affects men and women differently. Women generally are able to tolerate more pain, are much more open in conversations about the effects of pain, and are better able to cope with pain than men.

Here are a few different examples of knee pain that we frequently hear about:

> "I feel something moving in my knee, but I can live with it. It must mean that I am getting old, and I just have to get used to it."
> "My knee is not that bad. I sometimes feel the pain when I wake up."
> "Every time I bend down to tie my shoes, my knee gets so painful that I can barely walk at all afterward."

These are examples of different degrees of pain, from mild to potentially severe.

It is important to understand that even if your knee is only "bothering" you and not preventing you from performing your daily activities or sport, there is still a lingering problem that you need to take care of before it becomes worse. *Do not ignore your pain.* This is by far the most important rule to follow, if not in this chapter, then in this book.


## CAN MEDICATIONS HELP MY KNEE PAIN?

Yes, medications prescribed by your doctor can definitely help to relieve your knee pain. But medication is only a part of the game plan to fix your knee and keep it healthy and happy. Also, medications can produce some side effects, so speak to your doctor before taking anything. It is much better to have an experienced team around you than to try things on your own. It is also important to find a doctor who has some expertise with knee problems. Your family doctor might refer you to an orthopedic specialist of the knee as well as a physical therapist, osteopath, chiropractor, or other allied health professionals that could help.

Don't be afraid to get a second opinion about your condition if you are not sure about the diagnosis or if the medication is not working. This is especially important if you are being considered for surgery. Once the doctor has given you a diagnosis, some of the medications or treatments may include the following.

### Cortisone Shot

Some people ask about cortisone shots. What do they do exactly?

Cortisone shots are injections specifically in joints, like your knee. They have a corticosteroid medication and a local anaesthetic. Cortisone shots are normally performed in the doctor's office. They are supposed to help relieve pain and inflammation in your knee due to tendonitis or bursitis around the knee joint area. Typically, cortisone shots are used when other treatments—such as physical therapy or ice, heat, medication, and electrical modalities—are not helping.

For knee pain, cortisone is normally injected in a specific area of the knee to help understand if the limited range of motion is coming from the pain or from weakness. If the anesthetic relieves the pain and allows you to bend and straighten your knee properly, then the problem is probably some form of knee tendinitis or ligament strain.

After you receive your cortisone shot and the anesthetic wears off four to six hours later, you might feel some discomfort for a few days. Then corticosteroid in the cortisone shot should begin to kick in and relieve the pain and inflammation one or two days later. I have seen in my practice that cortisone shots can provide relief from inflammation and pain for several weeks or even more. But improvement varies: with other patients, it might be much less, like a week; and with some people, a cortisone shot might not help at all.

The maximum number of cortisone shots given is three to four shots. The number is limited due to the potential side effects of the medications. In addition, having multiple cortisone injections in the same area can weaken your quadriceps or other knee tendons. Your doctor may wait up to two months before giving another cortisone shot. If the first cortisone shot does not work, a second one may be given to ensure that it was given at the right spot. There are some side effects with cortisone shots, which include:

- increased pain the first few days after the injection;
- degeneration of the tendon in question;
- a change in skin color;
- infection at the site of injection (rare); and
- elevated blood sugar levels for those with diabetes.

Because of the injection, your quadriceps, hamstring, or other tendons may be a bit weaker than normal, so no strengthening exercises should be done for a couple of days afterward. You also should avoid contact sports after a cortisone shot, because you might further damage your knee.

Your allied health practitioner can use many different types of treatments from ultrasound to shockwave therapy, iontophoresis to interferential current, and everything in between.

**Medications**

If your doctor sees that you are suffering pain from your knee trauma, arthritis, or any other condition, he may prescribe medication. The doctor determines—based upon the symptoms that you present and your medical history—a treatment specifically for you.

*Topical Creams*

Analgesics are topical creams for pain that are rubbed into the area that hurts, whether a painful muscle, ligament, or tendon. There are different types of over-the-counter creams that ease pain. Some creams may contain salicylates, the same ingredient found in aspirin. When absorbed into the body, it helps decrease the pain, especially with joints close to the skin like your knee.

Another type of cream creates something called a "counterirritant" effect, tricking the brain into feeling the minor irritation or cooling sensation on the skin and forgetting to send the pain signal from your knee to your brain.

The last type of cream that I discuss here is creams that contains capsaicin, the ingredient found in hot chili peppers. Capsaicin is also one of the most effective ingredients for topical pain relief. It creates a feeling of warmth on your skin, because it heats up your skin and blocks the chemical that sends pain signals to your brain. You may need to apply these creams for a few days or up to a couple of weeks, according to the instructions on the package, before you notice reduced pain.

### NSAIDs

NSAIDs, which stands for nonsteroidal anti-inflammatory drugs, are among the most common pain relief medicines in a drugstore. Some of the more common brand names are aspirin, Advil, Motrin, and Aleve. In order to understand how NSAIDS work, you have to understand what causes the inflammation and pain first. Two types of COX enzymes—COX-1 and COX-2—create prostaglandins in the cells that promote inflammation and pain. NSAIDs block the COX enzymes from making prostaglandins, which reduces pain. I believe that NSAIDs play an important role in the treatment of knee pain and are not used to "mask" the pain, as some suggest. NSAIDs are another piece of the puzzle to healing your knee.

### Acetominophen

Acetominophen, which most of us know as Tylenol, has no anti-inflammatory components, so it is not part of the NSAID family, but it may help in some cases, especially if a person has a sensitive stomach and the NSAIDs cause too much discomfort in the stomach lining. According to the latest research, acetaminophen does not work to relieve the pain in individuals with osteoarthritic knees or hips.

## Ice

So, what can you do about the pain until you can get an appointment to see your doctor or physical therapist? There's a simple answer to this question, and it's amazing how many people in pain refuse to accept it: the solution is ice. What you want to do is numb the pain. Yet for some reason this seems counterintuitive to many people.

So why is ice better than heat when you are in pain? This is a very popular question, and I'll do my best to explain. Ice is an anti-inflammatory agent, just like Advil or aspirin. It reduces inflammatory activity from occurring at the injury site. Heat, however, is an inflammatory agent.

You want to decrease inflammation as much and as quickly as you can from the site of the pain, not increase it. Ice has been shown to be better than heat for any initial injury to the musculoskeletal system, especially during the first twenty-four to seventy-two hours.

So, what is inflammation? It's an automatic bodily response to an injury. Inflammation is like the body's garbage truck, removing waste products that are still around after an injury has occurred. Although inflammation is the first stage of the healing process and is necessary for your injury to eventually improve, the body tends to go overboard with inflammation production. This leads to problems if inflammation continue and swelling accumulates in the injured region. This swelling prevents normal oxygenated blood from reaching the injured tissues. If that occurs, it leads to a condition called secondary hypoxic injury, in which the cells are further injured or even die due to the lack of oxygen. When cell death occurs, the inflammatory process begins again. That's why ice (along with compression, elevation, and rest) is great for decreasing the inflammation, swelling, and hypoxia (lack of oxygen).

Ice can also reduce and even inhibit muscle spasms due to elevated pain levels. When ice is applied to a specific region, it lowers the temperature of that area and therefore decreases the amount of inflammation that the body produces in that region. Countless studies have shown that ice is the primary choice for relieving pain.

### Can I Ever Use Heat?

I do not recommend placing heat on an area that is painful, tender, or even very sore. With that said, there are times that heat can be beneficial. Sometimes, when you wake up in the morning and want to loosen up a part of your body, that might be a good time for using heat. (That's why taking a nice hot shower in the morning is so refreshing!)

By the way, the most efficient way to warm up a body part—drum roll, please—is exercise! Yes, that's right: exercise increases your body's core temperature more quickly (and safely) than other methods.

So once again, if you are looking to quickly loosen up your body, then heat is your answer. If you are feeling distress or discomfort, then go with the ice. You won't go wrong.

*Best Ways of Using Ice on an Injury*

There are a number of ways to "ice" an injury:

- place crushed ice in a Ziploc bag and wrap with a wet towel;
- wrap a bag of frozen peas or vegetables with a wet towel;
- use a commercial cold pack;
- experiment with pain-relief creams (such as Biofreeze cream);[
- try ice massage, gently rubbing the injured area in a circular manner with ice to numb it.

These are not the only methods of using ice. There are many other different ways, from cold whirlpool treatments, ice bucket treatments, all the way to different types of cold sprays.

*How do I do it?* Fill a sandwich-sized plastic bag—like a Ziploc—with ice cubes. Wrap the bag in a wet towel—yes, wet—and apply it to the point of pain. You can do this by lying down and placing the bag on your knee or by lying down with it under your knee. You can strap it to your knee with an elastic bandage, which you can obtain at your local drugstore or, perhaps, it is already in your medicine cabinet or first aid kit.

*Why a wet towel?* Because a wet towel is a far better conductor of cold than a dry towel and thus works far faster and more efficiently.

There are four stages of the pain-relieving process: cold, burning cold, aching, and numb. Numbness means you have frozen the pain, and you feel nothing. That is what you're shooting for. Once you reach this point, remove the icing apparatus.

*How long does it take to achieve numbness?* That, of course, varies from person to person, depending on the severity of the pain, the individual's pain threshold, and how well the icing apparatus is put together and applied. But as a general rule, it probably averages between ten and fifteen minutes for most people to achieve numbness.

If possible, ice the pain every couple of hours. Of course, this is a tall order for most working people, but try to do it at least twice a day—morning and night.

Then, be absolutely sure to avoid any kind of physical activity that could affect the knee. Certainly, do not return to the activity you were doing when you first felt the pain—whether it was playing tennis or reaching up to retrieve a book from an upper shelf. You may indulge in activities that don't affect the knee—go for a biceps curl if you like but no running, no jumping, no playing catch with the kids.

And whatever you do, see a licensed medical practitioner—even if the pain goes away. (It will likely come back.) It is important to receive a diagnosis of your injury, nontraumatic or traumatic, so you can move on.

Unless surgery is required, moving on focuses on physical therapy.

*When Not to Use Ice*

Do not use ice on your skin if you are suffering from any of the following.

*Cold allergies*: Ice allergies are extremely rare, affecting 1 to 2 percent of the population. Symptoms include hives, joint pain, and nausea. The removal of the ice bag helps clear this up.

*Reynaud's phenomenon*: This condition makes it much more difficult for blood to reach certain parts of your body because it makes the blood vessels under your skin tighten, which is called vasospasm.

This occurs in the fingers and toes. If that happens and no blood makes it to the fingers or toes, they turn blue and feel very cold. This is not a good sign. If you have not tried ice before, check the area frequently for this occurrence.

*Severe, large open wound*: Infections become the primary problem with open wounds, and you don't want to use anything that is not sterilized on them. Make sure large open wounds are covered with a sterile dressing.

*Decreased sensations to ice*: Anyone with a lack of sensation in a specific area should not use heat or ice in the affected region.

*Circulatory problems (i.e., hypertension)*: Cold should not be used on circulatory compromised regions of the body. Patients with circulatory problems can worsen their problems with ice, causing vasoconstriction in areas of the body that already experience nutritional deprivation, therefore exacerbating the situation.

*Diabetes:* Patients with diabetes have poor or decreased circulation to their extremities in varying degrees. When ice is placed on these compromised areas, local blood flow decreases. That's the last thing you want to do with an area that is not getting enough blood flow.

*When to Use Ice*

Ice can be an appropriate treatment in the following situations.

*Acute injury*: Ice should always be used during the first forty-eight hours after an acute injury. If heat is used at the injury site, inflammation increases, worsening the condition.

*Analgesia/pain relief:* Ice is always recommended when pain is involved. Ice reduces the velocity of nerve conduction and slows metabolism, reducing the cell's need for oxygenated blood, thus reducing additional cell death. If an area is numb, you won't feel the pain.

*Muscle guarding/spasm:* Studies have shown that ice is better for muscle spasms than heat. Ice creates a higher threshold for a nerve action potential or stimulus to occur, making a muscle contract. Heat has a lower threshold, creating spasms much more quickly.

There are definitely other excellent pain-reducing modalities that can be used for your injury. Please consult your doctor or health professional for any questions that you might have.

## MOVING ON—AND KEEPING THE PAIN AT BAY

Your physical therapist will clue you in on the operating principle of working on any muscle—namely, that you must achieve range of motion before strength, and you must achieve power before endurance. (At least, that's what the therapist *should* tell you; if he or she suggests strengthening exercises first, change therapists.) The theory behind this is simple and obvious: you don't want to strengthen the impairment of limited range of motion or you run the risk of locking in that limit. So the first aim of the knee-fixing process is achieving full range of motion. The process starts out easy, may proceed slowly, and often requires patience.

Of course, like Kayla, everyone wants to get back into their sport or activity quickly. But the truth is that there is no precise way to predict with any certainty how long it takes an individual to regain his or her full range of motion. Each case is different. Your therapist will ask to see some simple movements as a way to gauge the degree of flexion or extension—that is, the degree of bending and straightening—you may be missing. He or she may ask you to bend your knee as much as you can and then judge, for example, that you're "missing" 30 degrees of flexion and assign exercises that help you regain full flexion. How long it takes to do that depends on your age, your diligence in doing the exercises, your pain threshold, and more.

## THE "OVERDOING IT" DELUSION

Too much diligence can be as bad as too little. Al held to the belief that more is better. When his therapist assigned range-of-motion exercises once a day, Al instantly assumed that doing them three times a day would get him better three times faster. Morning, afternoon, and night, he kept at it for a week. By day eight, he was in so much pain from overworked muscles that he could barely bend his leg at all. Al could only wait till the spasms subsided and the pain disappeared before starting again from scratch. This time, he did it properly, patiently, and exactly as his therapist prescribed.

Not until range of motion has been solidly achieved should you attempt any kind of strengthening exercise. Physical therapists typically define "solidly achieved" as 70 to 80 percent of full range of motion as the absolute minimum for initiating strengthening exercises. Ideally, I recommend waiting till 100 percent of full range of motion has been achieved, but at the very least, I would suggest that you don't want to start the strengthening process until you have 80 percent of full range of motion. It isn't just that you run the risk of more pain, you also run the risk of real damage.

A regular patron at the gym where I work—I'll call him Salim—is a case in point. Tall with a powerful physique, Salim looks more like a bodybuilder than like a production executive in an entertainment company, which is what he is—an appearance stoked by the weight-lifting exercising to which he is partial. "No knee exercises at all till the pain is virtually gone," I advised him. "If you must work out"—and Salim shows up at the gym just about every day—"stick to exercises that work your upper body muscles. But don't do anything that affects or uses the knee. Certainly no running or jumping. It would really endanger your recovery."

Salim stayed away from the gym for a week. Then I noticed him on the jogging track and later taking a spin class on a stationary bike. Fine. I wasn't at work a few days later when Salim passed by the weight room at the gym and decided, in his own words, that he would do "just a couple of sets of light squats." It would be "no big deal," he thought. "Nobody will even know. It should be okay."

It was on the third rep of his second set that he heard the rip in his knee. Salim screamed. A guy on the next bench sat up and grabbed the weight out of Salim's hand as he cradled the leg against the floor. The doctor later confirmed that Salim suffered a complete muscle tear of his quadriceps and scheduled him for surgery the following week.

Surgery is the last thing you want. The bottom line? Listen to your pain, and do what your therapist tells you—no less and no more.

## HOW EATING RIGHT AND
## DIFFERENT TYPES OF THERAPY CAN HELP

It's no secret that eating healthy helps to make and keep your muscles stronger. It also helps injured muscles get stronger more quickly. You do not need a special diet to make your muscles stronger. Eating a balanced diet provides all the energy you need to go through your day. Keep in mind that irritation or inflammation of a joint, muscle, or tendon can slow down the healing process of the area. Therefore, some foods aid specifically in the healing of the tendons, just like exercise or massage.

As discussed earlier, tendons are extensions from muscles that attach on bones. They are made from dense connective tissue, which feels like a cord when you touch it through your skin. Because tendons have limited blood supply and are always working and under constant tension, it is difficult for them to repair quickly when a strain or tear has occurred.

Foods that have high active enzymes can provide a jolt that the tendons need and help them with the healing process. Examples of these super-foods are pineapple and papaya. These two foods have specific enzymes (called bromelain and papain) that are very active in the bloodstream and can contribute to helping the body heal the injured tendon more quickly.

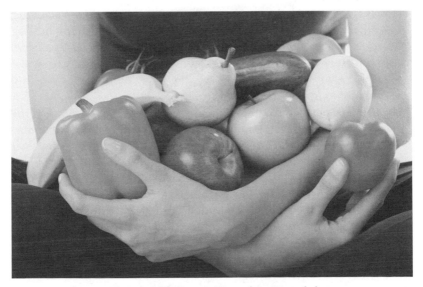

Fruits and Vegetables. *Kzenon. Image from Bigstockphoto.com*

Another important food contributor that aids in healing is any food that has vitamin C in it. The reason why vitamin C is so great is that it helps with the production of collagen, which is the most abundant in the tissue of a tendon. Great foods that contain vitamin C include broccoli (now you know why mom was right!), berries, oranges and other citrus fruits, tomatoes, peppers, brussels sprouts, and spinach.

Vitamin E is another great antioxidant that can help reduce inflammation. It is a fat-soluble vitamin and having too much of it can become toxic, so please don't overdo it. It is best to take vitamin E in food rather than a supplement. Vitamin E works together with vitamin C to create the formation of collagen. Vitamin E is interesting because it can be absorbed only if there is adequate fat in your diet. You can find vitamin E in such foods as nuts, seeds, avocados, and green leafy vegetables. Other vitamins and minerals that also can contribute to improving tendon health is vitamin B6, manganese, and zinc.

Tendons have quite a bit of calcium in them; therefore, eating foods that are rich in calcium can have a positive effect in the healing of the tendons. Milk products, as we all know, have plenty of calcium in them; fermented milk products like yogurt or buttermilk can also help.

There are also some nondairy foods that have a lot of calcium in them. My absolute favorite is salmon, as well as sardines, spinach, peas, broccoli, brussels sprouts, and bok choy. Basically, any food that is high in collagen or any other component of connective tissue is good for tendon healing. Therefore, meat is another good source, but fish and poultry is even better because there is much more connective tissue in them. It has been also shown that soup with joint or bone tissue—for example, pho, which is Asian tendon soup—is also a good choice.

Believe it or not, some juices can make tendons heal more slowly. Fruit juice is very high in sugar, and high blood sugar can increase inflammation. I suggest that you refrain from drinking juice, as it does not help with the nourishment of the body after a strain or sprain of a tendon. What I do recommend, however, is vegetable juices, especially cold juicing. This actually preserves the active enzymes found in the vegetables and still provides the concentrated nutrients. I also highly suggest drinking a lot of water during the day, approximately eight cups per day as a guideline.

Viscosupplementation is a popular injection treatment of hyaluronic acid, sometimes called Synvisc, which lubricates the joint to reduce knee pain and increase mobility. Basically, it acts like the synovial fluid that we naturally produce in our knees. A series of three to five injections a week are done. These injections are sometimes helpful for the treatment of pain in individuals with osteoarthritis who have not previously responded to oral medication.

One of the best supplements for knee joints is glucosamine. This fatty acid is a part of cartilage and other components of the joints. Glucosamine helps rebuild the bones and prevent cartilage wear and tear. It also prevents inflammation of the joints and adjoining muscles.

Another popular supplement is chondroitin sulfate. When combined with glucosamine, it helps build the cartilage and prevents pain in the joints. If chondroitin sulfate and glucosamine are taken in conjunction as supplements for joint pain, the pain may abate and the joints may become stronger.

Arnica, a popular herbal remedy, has been proven to help treat tendon and joint pain. It is normally applied and rubbed into the injured area in the form of an oil. Arnica has shown to decrease swelling and inflammation and can reduce the amount of time it takes for the tendon to recover.

Rue is another herbal remedy that can be used to relieve pain related to your tendonitis or other muscle injuries. An anti-inflammatory component in rue has been shown to strengthen the capillaries in the body.

There's been a lot of talk about omega-3s in the news, and for good reason. Found in fish, omega-3 fatty acids have been found to increase the body's anti-inflammatory response to tendonitis as well as many more health benefits. I really like it and try to incorporate it into all of my food, whether as an oil supplement or in my salmon.

Finally, cayenne pepper, although primarily known as a food seasoning, can also cause blood vessels to expand. This can help the body increase blood flow, bringing more much-needed nutrients to the injured tendon area and promoting healing.

There are many other nutrients, like turmeric and quercetin, that have anti-inflammatory properties and can help with the healing. Make sure to check with your doctor before starting any regimen for healing.

## CAN ACUPUNCTURE HELP MY KNEE?

Acupuncture is an ancient traditional Chinese medicine, dating back more than three thousand years, which involves correcting over almost two thousand points in the body that are connected along pathways of energy, normally called meridians. The energy points are called qi or chi. These points on the body have larger concentrations of nerve sensations and blood vessels than other parts of the body. Stimulating these points is said to remove any blocks in the qi meridians, clearing the way for the energy to move through the body, and therefore helping the body heal itself. Acupuncturists quote the ancient saying, "There is no illness except stagnation, no cure, only the reestablishment of flow in the body." The pathways of energy or flow are unblocked by needles. In 1996, the FDA gave acupuncture its first U.S. seal of approval when it classified acupuncture needles as medical devices.[2] In the twenty years since, study after study indicates that, yes, acupuncture can work.

We all know that there are needles involved in acupuncture. They are super thin, disposable stainless needles that are inserted through the skin and then twisted in a pattern along the meridians. The particular pattern in which the needles are placed depends on the injury and the patient's symptoms. The needles are then left in for approximately thirty to forty minutes. Different people feel different sensations from acupuncture. Some might say that they felt a pricking sensation with some warmth or an aching feeling. Some people might experience a sense of calm and relaxation to the point of falling asleep, whereas others might experience an increase of energy in their bodies.

The way that acupuncture can help your knee or any other type of pain is by stimulating the release of opioids, which are painkilling chemicals, as well as stimulating adenosine in the body, which is a natural painkiller and anti-inflammatory component.

*What's the difference between acupuncture and cortisone shots?* It really comes down to location. When a cortisone shot is used, it is placed at the injured site, which causes some discomfort to the patient. Acupuncture needles are placed above and below the injury, therefore not aggravating the irritated area at all. Acupuncture is very effective for knee tendinitis and other painful injuries. In case you were also wondering, acupuncture is safe with very few side effects at all, if done correctly by a professional, licensed acupuncturist.

If you're thinking about getting acupuncture, there are some things to keep in mind:

- Acupuncture can be dangerous if you are using certain medications, have a pacemaker, are at risk of infection, have chronic skin problems, or are pregnant.

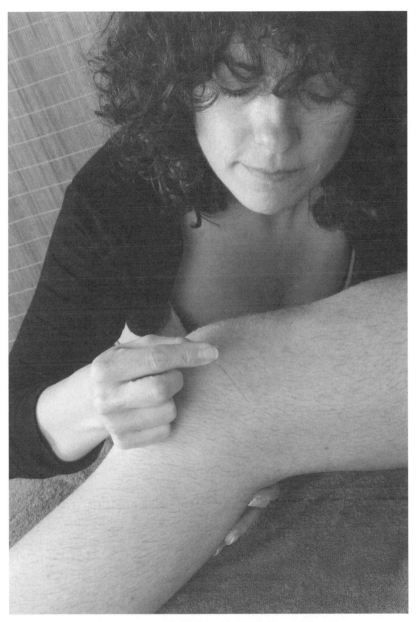

Knee Acupuncture. *Sylv1Rob1, image from Bigstockphoto.com*

- Check your acupuncturist's credentials. Most states require a professional license to practice. Acupuncturists must have proper documentation, just like physical therapists or medical doctors.
- Don't rely on disease diagnoses from acupuncture practitioners unless they're also licensed medical doctors. The American Academy of Medical Acupuncture can provide a referral list of doctors who practice acupuncture.
- Ask your medical doctor if acupuncture is a good option for your knee problems.

## WHAT ABOUT YOGA?

Yoga started thousands of years ago in India. It is a combination of exercise, stretching, controlled breathing, and meditation combined into one. When this form of exercise is done consistently and faithfully, it can reduce your pain and discomfort by stretching those areas of the body that are tight and inflexible. Yoga also does wonders for decreasing stress and tension levels in the body.

Sometimes, a yoga pose places additional stress on the joint, especially the most famous pose of all, the downward dog. This is a result of incorrect technique; for example, placing all the weight on the wrists instead of placing some of the weight on the hands. If you find that your fingers are lifting off the floor, this pose would probably give you some discomfort. Try placing your weight on your entire hand and gripping the mat with your fingers. This develops strength in your hands and fingers while at the same time taking stress off your joints, thereby decreasing the risk of developing tendonitis.

### How to Protect Your Knee While Doing Yoga

Try to not hyperextend your knees. Hyperextension, which is when your joint is loose enough that your leg can bend backward, often occurs in poses in which the legs are straightened, such as Trikonasana (triangle pose) and Paschimottanasana (seated forward bend). These positions can place pressure and strain on the back part of your knee capsule, hamstring, and calf muscles and tendons, as well as cause shearing, or excessive stretching force, on your ligaments. If your knees frequently hyperextend, it might be best to modify your movement. I suggest slightly bending your knees during the standing poses and distributing your weight evenly on your feet. In seated forward bends, place a rolled-up towel or your yoga mat behind the straightened leg or legs.

Placing your feet properly on the floor is a safe and effective way to increase power and strength on both sides of your leg and to avoid imbalances. When all the tendons and muscles are equally strong on both sides of your leg, your patella moves easily up and down the femur groove and the cartilage doesn't get worn out. Start by spreading out your toes evenly and distributing your weight equally throughout each foot, in every pose, even downward dog. If your feet are not properly placed on the floor and are out of alignment, you're going to feel it in your knees.

One of the biggest problems with some of these poses is aligning your knees properly. When performing a deep knee-bend pose, like Virabhadrasana II (warrior pose II) and Parsvakonasana (side angle pose), make sure that your bent knee is aligned over your ankle and your kneecap is in line with your second toe. Do not let your knee to go further in front of that toe or to move toward your first toe. Be aware of the position of your back foot, pressing it down evenly, while lifting from the arch of your front foot. It might at first be difficult to hold up the arch, but if you allow the arch on the inner part of your foot to drop, your knee will fall to the inside of your big toe, setting you up for several overuse symptoms and acute knee injuries.

Another useful trick is to listen to your knees. Sometimes, when you are in class and really into the movements, you won't feel the sensation or the feedback that the knees are giving you. Only later when the class is over will you start to feel the soreness and pain that results from not paying attention to your position. If you feel sore or achy when you come out of that bent-knee pose, you may have worked your knees too hard, and you should pay more attention to how deep you are bending.

Getting stronger through balancing exercises is something to work on. Poses that require balancing, especially the ones in which you must move in space while holding a bent standing leg such as Garudasana (eagle pose), really help. It has been shown that balancing while moving the rest of your body strengthens and protects your knees against future problems. This is because the poses train not only the muscles themselves, but also the nerves in coordinated movements, creating a better functional alignment of your hips, knees, and ankles, helping them work in unison.

If you perform seated asanas in your yoga program, experiment with props that might be lying around. In Virasana (hero pose), try bringing

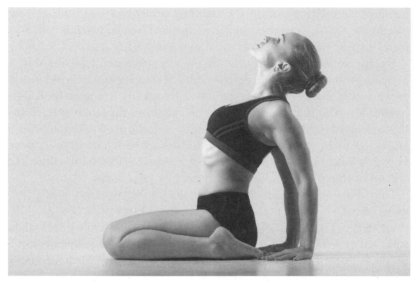

Hero Pose. *Fizkles, image from Bigstockphoto.com*

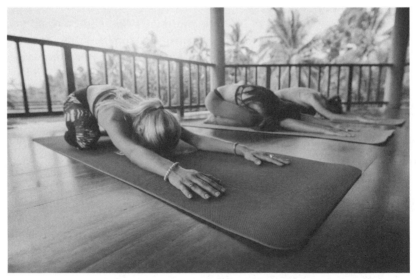

Child Pose. *Ammentorp image from Bigstockphoto.com*

your seat up higher by using some towels or a block. Any time the knees are in a deep knee-bend position, such as in Balasana (child's pose) or Marichyasana III (pose dedicated to the sage marichi III), try placing a rolled-up washcloth or face towel in the back of the knee, as far into the knee pit as possible before bending the joint, to decrease or even eliminate pressure in the knee.

Always warm up your body and joints before starting the poses. You can try warming up your hips with some hip openers or stretches like Baddha Konasana (bound angle pose) and Gomukhasana (cow face pose). Getting the big joints like your hips ready and warm takes some of the pressure off the smaller joints like the knee and ankles.

*Yoga Positions*

Some yoga poses that can help decrease or even alleviate knee pain follow.

*Supported warrior pose*: Standing in front of any available wall, place your hands on the wall, a shoulder-length distance apart. Place your left foot closer to the wall so that your toes are partially touching it, or at least stretched forward. Extend your right arm along the right leg and your left

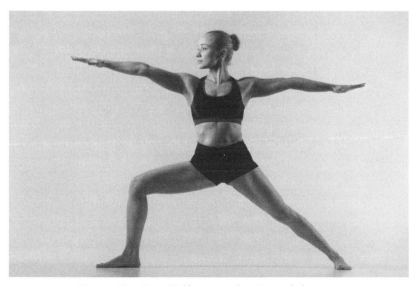

Warrior Two Pose. *Fizkles, image from Bigstockphoto.com*

arm along the left leg. Move your right foot two steps back and slightly bend your left knee. Try holding your breath for about fifteen seconds or so, and then stretch your left leg to repeat the exercise on the other side.

*Makrasana*: Sit down on your yoga mat or the floor. Slowly and gradually fold your legs gently into a lotus position. Use your fingers to hold the big toes of your feet and, while holding the same position of your lower limbs, try to lie on the floor by extending your back.

Touch the ground with your head, hold the position for a few seconds, and sit back in the original position. It can take some practice, but it really works!

*Tadasana*: This pose helps to relax your body and nourish the knee area. All you have to do is to stand up straight and place your feet firmly on the ground.

Keep your back muscles straight and maintain slow and steady breathing, focusing on breathing in from your nose and breathing out from your mouth. It takes time to master the breathing, but once you get it, you will feel the difference.

*Veerasana*: Start by placing both your knees and your hands on the ground, similar to a cat pose position. Slowly sit back and bend your legs

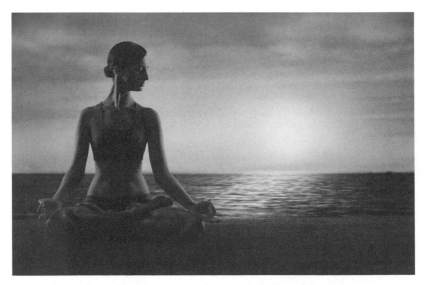

Makrasana Lotus Pose. *Inarik, image from Bigstockphoto.com*

inward. Next, fold your hands and position your wrists on your stomach. Take a deep breath and focus on relaxing your muscles and tendons, concentrating on your breathing.

*Triangle pose*: While standing up straight and maintaining your balance, stretch your right arm in the air, while at the same time stretching your left hand toward the ground. Hold the position for three to five seconds if possible, then slowly let go. Then, change sides and stretch the right hand toward the ground and the left arm in the air.

Done properly and consistently, the triangle pose stretches your adductor, or groin muscles, hamstrings, calves, shoulders, chest, and spine. It also strengthens your legs, knees, ankles, abdominals, obliques, and back.

*Camel yoga pose or ustrasana*: Start by kneeling down on the floor so that both your thighs are perpendicular to the floor. Place your shins on the floor and move your hands slowly to your pelvis. Then try to lean backward as much as you can and very slowly and carefully move your hands to your heels. Try holding the position for about three to five seconds and let it go.

If you find it difficult to keep your thighs perpendicular to the floor, try tilting the thighs backward individually as you touch hand to heel, using

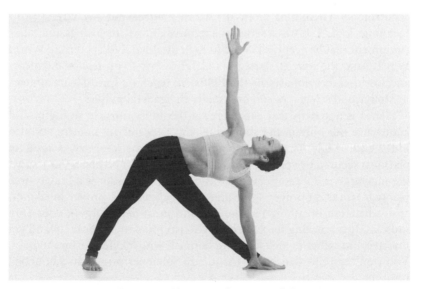

Triangle Pose. *Fizkles, image from Bigstockphoto.com*

either the left or right side limbs. Press each thigh back into perpendicular position before joining the opposite hand and heel.

If you cannot touch your feet without compressing your lower back, turn your toes under and raise your heels. Keep your head and neck in a neutral position, trying not to strain your neck or compress your throat. Try to work your way up to holding the position for thirty seconds, focusing on your breathing pattern.

This is a more advanced yoga pose that helps with knee stiffness and improves flexibility.

These yoga poses are helpful in alleviating knee pain and discomfort by strengthening and stabilizing the knee joint. However, if you experience undue pressure, stress, or strain in any part of knee joint, stop the exercise and try alternative poses to prevent any injury.

## SHOULD I DO PILATES?

Pilates is a form of exercise developed in the early 1900s by Joseph Pilates, a physical culturist from Germany who believed in the mind-body connection. We know now how true that is. After studying different forms of exercise and fitness, he developed a method of exercise that he called "contrology" (stemming from the word *control* and the Greek word meaning "logic"). It was a series of exercises done with springs and other equipment that he eventually used to help disabled soldiers during World War I. After the war, he started to teach his style to professional dancers and world-class gymnasts. By the 1980s, his teaching spread from athletes to Hollywood celebrities and eventually the general public.

Pilates is a system that can increase flexibility, muscle strength, and endurance not only in the abdominals, as is popularly known, but also in the entire body. The most famous apparatus, the reformer, is a rolling platform secured by springs. It is unique in that you lie down flat against the machine. It does not compress the spine, because it is a gravity-free plane. It works on proper spine and pelvis alignment, proper inhalation and exhalation breathing techniques, and most definitely on your core muscles. It is amazing for someone who isn't looking to bulk up and get massive, but rather to look lean and defined, with a killer posture to boot. You won't see elite dancers or Cirque du Soleil performers in a hunched position.

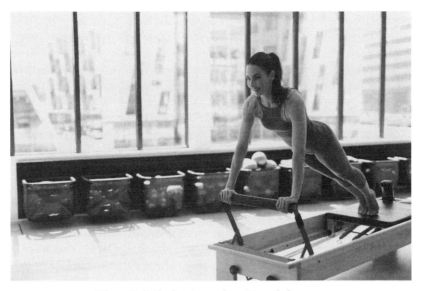

Pilates. *Belinda_bw, image from Bigstockphoto.com*

Although Pilates often relieves problems such as knee pain, realignment and relief from chronic knee ailments take time and consistent effort.

If you have tight or inflexible quadriceps and poor knee flexion and extension, Pilates can cause stiffness and soreness in the knee joints. If an underlying problem exists when you begin Pilates, you're more likely to feel soreness of the knees during a standing workout that requires squatting rather than lying down on the reformer.

The footwork on the bar exercises is the perfect series of exercises for improving strength and alignment of the entire lower body, from feet to hips. As one leg stretches, the other leg strengthens, remaining rigid. It is like stationary one-leg calf raises, but in a recumbent position.

Side-lying movements, normally done in a standing position, work the abductors and lateral hip while flexing and extending the knee.

There is a component of the reformer machine in which you can place your feet in straps. There are a wide variety of exercises, and they are fun to do. These exercises are excellent for strengthening and stretching adductors (inner thighs) and hamstrings, as well as hip flexors.

"Bridging" on the reformer is extremely effective in strengthening the gluteal muscles and the hamstrings, as well as stabilizing the back of the knee. This is one of my favorite exercises to show patients—especially women—who have stronger quads and weaker hamstring and glute muscles.

The exercise options for the reformer are endless. If you took a private reformer class in your area with a qualified instructor, he or she would probably perform a gait and postural analysis to indicate where your muscle imbalances lie and why you keep injuring your knees. Once this imbalance has been identified, a specific program is created to stretch out the tight muscle groups and strengthen the weaker muscle groups, thus restoring your knees to their pre-injury function.

The original six principles of Pilates training include the following.

*Centering*: According to the Pilates method, the way to control your arms and limbs is to develop your core, which is the center of your body. Referred to as your "powerhouse" area, all movements should start from this area and move outward. This makes all other movement much more efficient and much less energy draining. The secret to developing this powerhouse region is to try to maintain a neutral pelvis while doing the exercises.

*Concentration*: In order for Pilates training to be successful, you must have intense concentration and focus on what you are doing. This is why I am a big believer in one-on-one Pilates training. Normally in a Pilates studio, it is quiet. No blaring music, no human distractions. It is just you and the instructor. Of course, there are two-on-one classes and even group classes, but it is not the same experience. The instructor cannot be everywhere trying to spot if anyone is cheating (and there will be times that you yourself do not know that you are cheating). The best way of getting your money's worth is to have an instructor with you to correcting your movements. You will feel a big difference. You are so focused on what your teacher is trying to get you to do that there is no way for distractions to interfere with training.

*Control*: With concentration comes control.

*Flow:* Pilates always aims for an elegant flow of proper movement through specific precision. Once that high level of precision has been attained, then movements smoothly flow from one exercise to another, which builds stamina and strength. Therefore, Pilates builds smooth, controlled, flowing exercises from your strong core.

*Precision*: Pilates teachers emphasize precision to their students, which is to focus on doing one perfect movement rather than many imperfect ones. The reason for this is to make these super-hard exercises become easy and natural for you. This also carries forward in the grace and economy of movement in your everyday life.

*Breathing*: This is the principle that newcomers say is the hardest to master: proper breathing. Pilates believed that full inhalation and exhalation was the key to cleansing the body and feeling invigorated.

Pilates always stated that full-forced exhalation was the key to complete exhalation. Pilates breathing is breathing deeply into your back and the sides of your rib cage. When you breathe out, contract your deep abdominals and pelvic floor muscles. Maintain this position as you continue to inhale. It is important to combine your breathing with the exercise movements that you are performing. Above all, Pilates wanted his clients to learn how to breathe properly.

## SUMMARY

- Pain is a signal; pay attention to it.
- Apply ice to pain and work through the four phases of the pain relieving process: from cold to burning cold through aching to numbness, which is the goal.
- Full rest from knee activity is advised until pain is gone.
- The exercise therapy progression is to achieve range of motion before strength and power before endurance.
- Ideally, you should regain range of motion fully—100 percent—before initiating strengthening exercises, but at the very least, regain 80 percent of your range of motion first.
- Always put ice on an injury, never heat.
- The best way to apply ice to an injury is to place crushed ice in a Ziploc bag with a wet towel wrapped around it.
- If you are not sure whether to use ice or heat in your situation, always choose ice.
- If using ice for the first time, make sure you do not have any contraindications.
- Pilates is a system that can increase flexibility and muscle strength in your knees without increasing compression and stress.
- Yoga is a combination of exercise, stretching, controlled breathing, and meditation combined in one. When this form of exercise is done

consistently and faithfully, it can reduce your pain and discomfort by stretching areas that are tight and inflexible. It also does wonders to decrease everyday stress and tension in your body.

- Acupuncture unblocks the qi meridians and clears the way for the energy to move through the body, which helps the body to heal itself.

# 4

# The Knee Shop

Dear Baby Jesus, take the pain in my legs from yesterday's workout.

—Will Ferrell

Doing exercises isn't fun. No one really likes doing them. We'd rather watch TV, go for a walk, or do something else rather than doing rehabilitation exercises or going to a gym. But doing exercises is the number-one way of getting stronger and more flexible and improving balance. Exercise also decreases or eliminates what you are trying to rid yourself of: pain. Creating a balanced program of stretching, strengthening, and balance exercises is what this book is all about.

I am a firm believer that through proper exercise, hard work, and dedication to your program you can fix most knee injuries. This is exercise as therapy—a Greek word meaning "cure" or "healing"—something that I'm sure sounds attractive.

In the last chapter of this book, I offer more advanced exercises that you can do primarily in a gym setting, with specific routines you can practice for a lifetime to keep your knee strong and flexible, reducing stiffness and outright pain. This is exercise for prevention of future knee injuries, and it is just as important as and even more useful than exercise as therapy.

Whatever end result you seek, whether to fix what has gone wrong or to maintain a sound, strong, stable condition in your body, exercise exists in a context—in its own frame of reference. It is essential to understand the parameters of that context before you undertake any exercise program, and that's what this chapter is about.

Specifically, the context consists of three things: the warm up, the way we count or measure exercises—as sets of repeated movements separated by rest—and the stretching that ideally takes place after the exercises. Here are the whys and wherefores of each.


## THE WARM UP

We take warm ups for granted and sometimes neglect them altogether. That can be a costly mistake. The purpose of a warm up is to loosen up your knee—and your body in general—so that you don't reinjure what you've spent so much time and effort trying to fix. In fact, research has shown that a proper preventative warm up among soccer players decreased injuries by improving the strength in their legs.

When you warm up a muscle, it means precisely that: raising its temperature. Raising the temperature in turn means that you can contract that muscle and the surrounding area more forcefully and efficiently. The warm up also drives oxygenated blood into the knee area, which in turn raises your blood pressure just a bit, thus also increasing your heart rate. This is a good thing. When you increase your heart rate, you get the heart pumping the maximum amount of oxygen throughout the body while at the same time eliminating the waste products created by the work your muscles have done up to that point.

A great warm up helps you not only to feel better, but it also improves your workout, making it more efficient. A motivation and incentive for warming up properly might be knowing that it can improve your squat or deadlift, for example, making it even better than if you didn't warm up.

Some people believe that biking for five minutes or arm curling weights a couple of times means that they have properly warmed up, but that's where problems can start. Beyond not getting yourself loosened up fully and not stimulating your nervous system—which in turn stimulates your muscles, getting them ready for more strenuous exercise—there's another problem. Neglecting the problem areas around your legs like weak glutes and hips, poor abdominal core, and poor spine mobility can cause injuries, even among athletes. By not warming up, you are asking for anterior knee pain, hamstring pulls, or even back pain. Try to bulletproof your body instead of setting yourself up for failure.

A proper warm up doesn't just get you going: warming up can also extend your fatigue limit. When your body is ready for an intense workout, it can last longer than if you start cold. And, of course, a good warm up helps prevent pulling or overstretching muscles. Muscles that are warmed up before an intense activity are more pliable and loose. They can more easily absorb the forces the exercises exert upon them.

So think of the warm up as the pregame activity before the main show. In my view, your warm up routine should take about twenty minutes on average, depending on your needs and fitness level. Once you've completed your warm up and are primed and prepared, your muscles feeling toasty warm and eager to get to work, your heart, lungs, and nervous system on the mark and waiting for the starting gun, you are ready to begin your workout.

Avoid the pitfalls of poor warm ups and take a few minutes before every workout to prepare yourself, build more strength, and prevent injuries. Your knees will thank you.

## NUMBER COUNTING: REPS, SETS, AND REST PERIODS IN BETWEEN

Understanding reps, sets, and rest periods between them is important so that you can modify your workout in order to improve it. Changing the parameters of your workout creates new growth in the muscle tissues.

*Reps* is short for repetition. It refers to the number of times that you repeatedly perform any movement, whether a squat or a step up. Ten reps of squat mean that you squat down and stand up ten times. The lifting up plus the lowering down together count as a single repetition.

However, there's more to it than just an up-and-down motion, for both movements of a single repetition are important. Doing both of them properly is essential, both for getting all possible benefit from your exercise routine and for staying safe. Unfortunately, one phase of the rep tends to get all the attention while the second is typically neglected—in my view, with very serious adverse results.

Of the two phases of a single weight-training repetition, the concentric phase is the more difficult: it is the lifting or pulling motion in which the muscle gets shorter, and it should be done explosively—with proper form—in one to two seconds. That explosiveness is what recruits the maximum amount of muscle and tendon fibers in order to increase strength. The eccentric phase of the rep, the phase in which the muscle gets longer, follows. All too often, we apply little if any effort to this phase.

Instead, we let gravity take over and more or less allow the weight to drop in what is basically a wasted movement.

This is a mistake. The eccentric phase of the rep should not be wasted movement. In fact, I believe that a number of knee injuries could be avoided altogether if the eccentric phase of a repetition is executed properly and given the same attention as the concentric phase. Performing the eccentric phase in a slow and controlled manner, in three to four seconds, strengthens your muscles as they lengthen. It's the way that many professional and Olympic athletes train, both for sustained strength in every phase of every movement and to decrease the chance of injury.

The reason is simple: paying equal attention to both phases of a rep balances your muscles. In my view, balance is the single most important word in the entire physical therapy universe because it is the single most important thing a body can be. If you are balanced in strength from every direction, with proper flexibility and range of motion, you can avoid sports-related injuries. That's why doing the repetition correctly, attending to both its phases, is more important than the number of repetitions you do.

A set is the number of repetitions of the exercise you perform without stopping. If you lift a weight ten times then stop and take a break, that is a single set of ten repetitions. One way to determine the number of repetitions you should do is to push yourself to the point of momentary muscle failure—that is, continue doing reps while maintaining proper technique until you simply cannot do another rep. This is a good way to increase strength gains in your muscles.

Alternatively, most exercise programs such as the ones I present in this book set forth a goal for each exercise: a specific number of sets and reps advisable for maintaining strength and fitness through performing the particular exercise. As you will see, ten repetitions is a fairly common goal for a set, and when you see that an exercise program calls for "3x10" of a particular exercise movement, that means you're being asked to do three sets of ten repetitions: ten reps of the movement followed by a break, then another ten reps followed by another break, and another ten reps.

Three sets of ten reps is by no means the only program advised for an exercise routine, but it is the most commonly practiced and the mainstream methodology for weight training. Although in Olympic lifting or powerlifting, fewer sets and fewer reps with heavier weights are common, and some research suggests that one set of exercises might be as effective as three, but three sets of ten continues to be the norm, and I'll be using it as a goal for exercises in this book as well.

Why ten repetitions instead of four—or fourteen—and why three sets instead of six—or the one set that research claims may be just as effective? Let me explain. Different frequencies of repetition produce different results. Fewer repetitions—typically anything less than seven—affect muscle strength. More repetitions—say twelve to twenty—work the muscle's capacity for endurance rather than strength. Therefore, eight to ten repetitions is somewhere between strength and endurance, theoretically benefiting both: a low enough number of repetitions to boost endurance and develop stability while also high enough to increase strength and power. What you don't want to do is fewer repetitions with greater weight, because that raises the possibility of too much stress on the knee and doing more harm than good. We want your knee area to be as strong as possible, but we also want to do that as safely as possible.

Similarly, three sets with a rest break between each set constitute a solid middle ground: a sufficient number of reps to be effective without exhausting or straining the muscles.

Keep in mind that when working out, you should not be in pain while doing an exercise. If you feel pain, you need to change your routine. Either decrease the weight, rest longer, or do fewer sets. Working out should be enjoyable, not painful. When it is enjoyable, you keep doing it, and that's what will help you to realize amazing gains in a safe and effective way. And by the way, yes, people will notice that you look stronger and more muscular.

## STRETCH!

Often, stretching is not taken seriously. "I'll stretch later" or "I don't need it" are the excuses I hear sometimes. Stretching has always taken a backseat to strengthening, but it is important for your health and well-being, and it makes you feel good. It is one of life's pleasures and one of the best remedies for just about anything that ails you. Done properly and consistently every day, stretching is one of the best things you can do for yourself, and it's certainly the perfect way to end any exercise routine. Staying limber and flexible as you get older is a great idea, because it helps you move better.

For one thing, stretching is simply healthy for the body. Done regularly, stretching can help you maintain range of motion and flexibility throughout your lifetime, no matter your age. It counters the muscle-shortening effects of long hours sitting at a desk or of bad posture, and that means fewer and less acute aches and pains.

This is why I recommend stretching every day, even if only once a day. Of course, there are days when you simply cannot, but don't let the lapse continue—try to start up again the next day. You can stretch any time, day or night. After all, it's not as if stretching your body requires special equipment or clothing, nor does it take up a whole lot of your day, although it isn't something you can zip through.

The American College of Sports Medicine (ACSM) recommends stretching each of the major muscle groups for at least thirty to sixty seconds every time you stretch. Quick stretches of fifteen seconds or so simply do not give the muscle enough time for optimal lengthening. So what constitutes proper stretching? The truth is that there are many ways to stretch—at least half a dozen different techniques, each with its own name and purpose, from dynamic to ballistic to active isolated and more. The easiest and least complicated type of stretch is the static stretch. As the name implies, it's all about putting a muscle in a stretch position and holding it static for a period of time.

*Here's how*: Assume the stretch position for the muscle, begin the stretch, and when you feel a gentle pulling, stop pushing. Hold the position for at least sixty seconds, then slowly release. Rest for thirty to sixty seconds, then try it again.

The stretch can feel a bit uncomfortable, but it should not be painful. If you feel pain, stop immediately and decrease the pressure. Do not for a moment suppose that if you push harder, you'll get better results. The opposite is the reality: you might end up hurting yourself instead of giving yourself relief.

There should be no bouncing in static stretching. Bouncing is for ballistic stretching, and in my view, bouncing or moving too quickly in and out of a movement can cause injury.

I don't mind admitting that I normally listen to music on my headset while I do my stretches. It helps pass the time—both the time spent stretching and the breaks of at least sixty seconds that I give myself between stretches. Stretching makes me feel loose and full of energy, and I find that the feeling of well-being is best achieved when I do a stretch three times for thirty to sixty seconds, so that's what I typically recommend to my patients.

Warm up, the workout, the postworkout stretch: these are the elements of any exercise program, whatever its purpose. Our purpose is to get your knee better, so let's turn to that now.

Stretching after an exercise workout helps maintain range of motion and aids in preventing injury. Static stretching is recommended using a formula of three sets held for thirty to sixty seconds each with thirty seconds of rest between sets.

I believe that an exercise-based treatment is the number-one best and fastest way to heal most impairments of the knee, barring surgery. In this chapter, I discuss the most essential exercises that you need to help your knee. These strengthening and range-of-motion exercises will have a direct, positive benefit on the rapid rehabilitation of your knee. I will tell you how to perform the exercise in the proper form. These are by no means the only exercises that you can do to strengthen your knee, but these are the ones that I share with my patients on a daily basis. Now I want to share them with you—enjoy!

## RANGE-OF-MOTION (ROM) EXERCISES

The purpose of these range-of-motion or ROM exercises is to reduce stiffness in your knee, to increase flexibility, and to restore your knee's full range of motion, all of which is needed in order to perform your daily activities. If your knees feel stiff and painful, move them gently through their range of motion, just enough that you feel some tension or stretch without pain. Move slowly into the exercise without bouncing. Never force the movement. Make sure you breathe throughout the exercise: holding your breath won't help.

Perhaps the most important of all the points made here is to *stop* exercising if you experience extreme pain. It's possible that you might have gone too far into the movement.

### Heel to Behind

This is probably the range-of-motion exercise that everyone starts with to gain full knee flexion. Start by lying on your back, keeping your uninjured leg straight and your arms at your side. Take the heel of your injured leg and start sliding it toward your behind until you start to feel a slight discomfort or pull. Once you feel pulling, return your leg to the starting position.

*Your goal*: three sets of ten repetitions.

*What to watch out for*: Do not force the movement. It should not be painful. Do not do this with your shoes on but wear socks instead, as they slide the best.

**Assisted Knee Flexion**

This is an exercise that helps with knee flexion when you can't work your injured leg itself; the good leg helps you out. This specific exercise can be done once your knee can be at a right angle with the floor. While sitting, place your good foot in front of the bad or injured foot, and start to bring the good leg backward until you feel pulling in your injured knee. Hold the position for a count of one or two seconds, stretching the knee without pain, then slowly release, allowing your leg to return to the starting position.

*Your goal*: three sets of ten to twenty repetitions, holding for one to two seconds.

*What to watch out for*: Concentrate on relaxing the muscles of your affected leg when doing this exercise. It should be performed only within a pain-free range of motion. You should feel some contraction in your muscles but no sharp pain inside the actual knee joint. Do not continue this exercise if there is pain, swelling, or a significant increase in skin temperature (i.e., if skin becomes hot/warm to the touch).

Do not perform this exercise on a soft surface (i.e., a bed), because you will not achieve the desired results. Do not use quick, jerky movements while doing this exercise; it is intended to be performed in a slow and controlled motion. If you find that the edge of your chair limits the amount of flexion you can achieve comfortably, try this exercise on the edge of a table, which provides more freedom to dangle and move your leg.

**Prolonged Knee Extension**

After a severe knee injury or surgery, which has left the leg with excess scar tissue making it difficult to extend the leg fully, this exercise might be useful in restoring the full extension.

Sitting on a chair, place your foot on a stool or another chair in front of you. Leave the knee unsupported, allowing gravity to slowly start to pull the leg downward, thereby increasing extension. If you do not feel any pulling movement, you can place a small weight on your leg to help facilitate the extension. Hold the position for one to two minutes each time, and give yourself one-minute breaks in between sets.

*Your goal*: three sets of ten reps, holding for one to two minutes, resting for one minute in between sets.

*What to watch out for*: Some people overdo this exercise, holding the position for much longer than is recommended with the thought that more is better. All that does is create pain, soreness, and difficulty walking. Remember that success requires patience.

## Hip Internal Rotation Self-Stretching

The hips are very important to overall knee health, though they might not seem so to the casual reader. Limited hip internal rotation can be seen in people who have a "penguin" style of walk or whose feet fully turn to the outside when walking. This exercise brings your legmore toward the middle, helping with knee conditions like patellofemoral pain syndrome and chondromalacia.

Lying on the floor on your back, bend both of your knees, keeping them apart slightly wider than shoulder width. If you plan to internally rotate your right hip, then take your left ankle and place it on top of your right thigh. With your left ankle, start applying pressure to the outer or lateral part of your right thigh inward or toward the middle of your body. You will feel pressure on the inside of your hip. Hold the position for thirty to sixty seconds.

*Your goal*: three sets of ten reps, holding for thirty to sixty seconds, resting for one minute in between sets.

*What to watch out for*: If you don't feel pressure in your hip area with your knee at that angle, try slightly straightening your knee while continuing to apply pressure on your thigh. Again, stop when you begin to feel discomfort, not pain. If you can't maintain thirty to sixty seconds, that's OK. Hold the exercise as long as you can and gradually build up your tolerance over time.

## Hip External Rotation Self-Stretching

Although this deficit is seen less often than hip internal rotation, having good hip mobility is essential to optimal knee function and control.

Lying on your back, keep your knees bent, slightly wider apart than shoulder width. If you are working on the right hip, take your left foot and place it on your inner thigh just above your knee joint area. If you can't reach your right leg properly, move the leg closer so that your foot is firmly planted on the thigh. Slowly start pushing your right leg away from you without moving your right ankle. It must stay where it's at. This creates outside rotation, opening up your hips and probably stretching your groin in the process. Again, try holding the position for thirty to sixty seconds if possible.

*Your goal:* three sets of ten reps, holding for thirty seconds, resting for one minute in between sets.

*What to watch out for:* Don't try to push the leg too far and hurt yourself. Focus more on opening up the joint rather than stretching the groin. If you are stretching your groin *and* opening your hip, that's a good position in which to continue.

## STRETCHING EXERCISES

### Quadriceps Stretch

A lot of people who feel pressure or discomfort in their knees have tight or inflexible quadriceps muscles. If the quadriceps get tight, they can pull the kneecap out of position slightly, causing friction at the knee. If you find yourself sitting down for long periods of time, such as when you're watching a movie or taking a long airplane flight, and feel the need to extend your leg and release the pressure in the knee, your quads might need stretching.

There are many ways to stretch your quad muscles, but this is my favorite way to give the muscle a really good pull. To stretch your right quads, lie on your left side. Bring your left knee upward toward your head. It is not necessary to grab the knee with your other hand, just bring it as high as you can and leave it comfortably in that position.

Bend your right knee. Place your right hand on your right ankle. From this position, pull your knee back until you start to feel a stretch in your

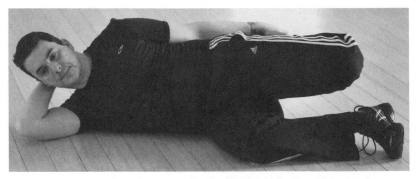

Quadriceps Stretch. *All photos in chapter 4 by the author.*

quads muscles. It should not be painful. Try holding the position for approximately one minute.

*Your goal*: three sets of ten reps, holding for one minute, resting for thirty seconds in between sets.

*What to watch out for*: The nonstretching leg is the secret to this exercise and the reason I prefer to do it lying on the side rather than standing up. If, instead of bending your nonstretching leg, you kept it straight, you would not get the same stretch. When your knee is brought up in the direction of your head, it locks the hips, not allowing them to move. This in turn won't allow you to "cheat" on your stretch, so you get the full benefit.

However, if you are outside and cannot lie down on the floor, the standing stretch is the next best thing. As long as you can visualize pushing the hip forward as you stretch, you should feel pulling in your quads.

There are many ways to do a quad stretch, so choose the best way for you—just be sure to hold the position for at least a minute or so. Research has shown that during the first fifteen seconds of a static stretch, the muscle fibers actually contract to protect themselves. After fifteen seconds or so, the muscle starts to loosen up. That's why holding a position for one minute or longer (I hold my position while listening to an entire song on my iPhone) gives you the best results, loosening your patella so that it can move around better and decrease pressure on your knee.

## Hamstring Stretch

Hamstring tightness is a common issue for people with knee pain. Stretching and loosening your hamstring not only reduces pressure on your knees, but because the hamstring is a muscle that passes through two joints, it also relieves pressure from your hips and back.

There are many ways to stretch your hamstring, but this is one of my favorites. It is best for those who do not have back pain.

Sitting with your feet in front of you, bend the leg you are not stretching so that the foot rests against the inner thigh of the leg that you are stretching. You don't need to jam your foot all the way to your groin, just place it comfortably on the inner thigh.

Place the leg that you want to stretch in front of you. With both hands on your knee or slightly above on your thigh, slowly start to bend forward, with your chest moving toward your leg, keeping your head straight, until you feel a pull in your leg. Hold that position for one minute.

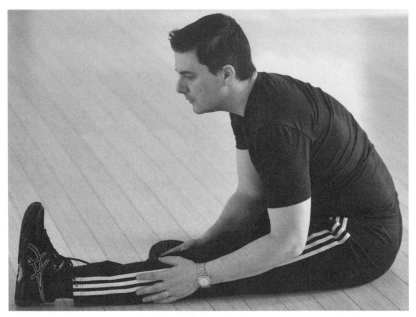

Hamstring Stretch.

*Your goal*: three sets of ten reps, holding for one minute, resting for thirty seconds in between sets.

*What to watch out for*: Many people try to reach for their feet. It's almost instinctive, but don't do it. It causes unnecessary strain on your back. It's better to reach forward with your body rather than with your head. If you want more of a stretch, then start by very slowly bringing your foot of your nonstretching leg toward you. Your hamstrings should pull a little more. Go for consistency, working on the stretch every day, moving just a little closer to your goal.

**Lying Down Hamstring Stretch**

If you experience back pain, this is another way to stretch your hamstring safely and effectively.

Start by lying on your back with your good knee bent. Place a towel around your ankle so that you can pull your leg up to stretch it. Slowly straighten your leg, still holding the towel, until you feel a stretch behind your leg. If you do not feel a stretch, slowly pull on the towel, bringing your injured leg closer to you. You should start to feel a pull in your hamstring area.

*Your goal*: three sets of ten reps, holding for one minute, resting for thirty seconds in between sets.

*What to watch out for*: Although it might be a natural tendency to lift the head up while doing this stretch, it also causes strain and discomfort in your neck. Keep your head down and focus on the hamstring stretch. Try to keep your body, face, neck, and shoulder muscles relaxed when performing this stretch.

## Glutes Stretch

Tight glutes often cause pain in the knees, hips, or back by slightly altering the position of the leg, causing an uneven distribution of forces through the knee. Keeping the glutes loose and supple decreases the stress on your knees.

This exercise can be done in a sitting position. Begin by sitting on the floor and putting both of your legs in front of you. Place the foot of the leg that you want to stretch on the side of your straight leg, so that your legs resemble the number four (or a backward four, depending on the leg

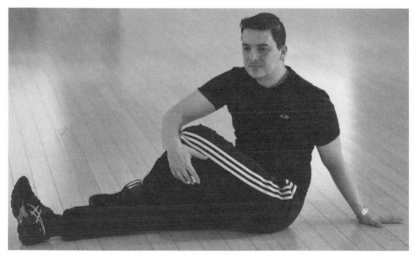

Glutes Stretch.

you're stretching). Keeping your back straight, pull the leg to be stretched toward your chest until you feel a good pull in the glutes area. Try holding this position for one minute before letting go.

*Your goal*: three sets of ten reps, holding for one minute, resting for thirty seconds in between sets.

*What to watch out for*: Keep your back straight without twisting. Pull your leg toward you until you feel a good stretch (but no pain). There are other variations of this exercise, but my patients get the best results with this particular one.

## Piriformis Stretch

This is another simple stretch that can loosen up your hips.

Lying on your back, bend both knees while keeping your feet flat on the floor. Place the outside of the foot of the leg that you want to stretch against the lower thigh of the other leg. Slide both hands around your thigh, one from the outside and one from the inside, connecting your hands together. Grip behind your thigh and pull the knee toward your chest. You should feel a stretch in the buttock. Hold this position for one minute or so, keeping your back flat.

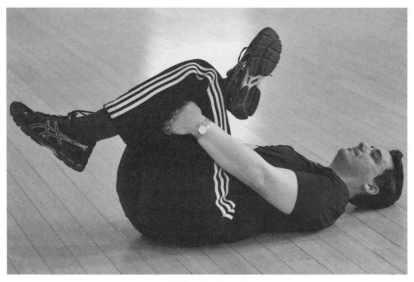

Piriformis Stretch.

*Your goal*: three sets of ten reps, holding for one minute, resting for thirty seconds in between sets.

*What to watch out for*: Your eventual goal is to bring your knee to your chest. It might sound crazy, but it is possible through daily practice.

## Hip Flexor Stretch

This is a stretch that opens your hips, allowing your knees and hips to move together better. If you have tight hips, you usually have weak, overstretched glutes and hamstrings. The best way to help yourself is to balance out the muscles in your legs, making the front and back flexible and equal in strength.

Kneel on one knee with your back leg being the one you are about to stretch.

Keep your body straight and squeeze your glutes as hard as you can. Then, keeping your glutes tight, your body straight and tall, and your head facing forward, lean forward at the hips, holding about thirty seconds or so, with the eventual goal of about sixty seconds.

*Your goal*: three sets of ten reps, holding for one minute, resting for thirty seconds in between sets.

*Things to look out for*: If it hurts to kneel, try placing a yoga mat on some towels under your knee. That should cushion the force and allow you to hold the position. If you find yourself losing your balance while performing this stretch, try holding a stick, such as a broom or a hockey stick, on the side of the leg that you are stretching. That should balance you out better.

## Groin or Adductor Stretch

The groin is commonly a tight area on many people. The groin or adductor area starts in the hips and extends all the way down to the upper inner side of the knee.

My favorite way to stretch this area is as follows. Sitting down on the ground, place the soles of your feet together with your knees pointing outward. This position has been referred to as the "butterfly" position. Grab your feet with your hands. Slowly lean forward until you start to feel a stretch in your groin region. Some people prefer to bring their head toward their knees to get a better stretch, and that's OK if it helps. Another variation is to place your hands on your inner thighs and push down rather than holding your feet and leaning forward. It can be a challenge for my patients to push down hard enough to get the most out of the stretch, but if you do it this way and get a decent stretch, then by all means go ahead. Always use the technique that works best for you.

*Your goal*: three sets of ten repetitions, holding for one minute, resting for thirty seconds in between sets.

*What to watch out for*: Sometimes people go too far with this exercise and end up pulling the groin that they are trying to stretch. Please ease into it, increasing your range of motion on a day-to-day basis. Eventually, it will loosen up, and remain loosened without injury.

## Calf Stretch

Some people wonder why calf stretching is important in alleviating knee pain. The calves should be involved primarily with ankle problems, not knee problems. In the calf region, there are two muscles: the soleus and the gastrocnemius, or gastroc for short. The soleus muscles connect from the Achilles tendon to the tibia, whereas the gastroc muscle starts at the Achilles tendon, but attaches above the joint line of the knee. Therefore, a tight calf can cause difficulty in fully extending the knee without knee pressure. Therefore, stretching out the calf is important.

Stand in front of a wall, with your good leg in front and the bad or injured leg in the back, keeping the heel of the back foot firmly planted on the floor. Place your forearms on the wall so that you can be in a more comfortable position to perform the stretch. Start bending the front leg forward until you start feeling a stretch in your back leg. Try holding the position for about a minute or so.

*Your goal*: three sets of ten reps, holding for one to two minutes, resting for thirty seconds in between sets.

*What to watch out for*: Make sure that your feet are pointed forward toward the wall. Sometimes, there's a tendency to turn your foot inward, stretching a different part of your calf muscle without stretching the calf heads equally. Also, make sure that your heel is flat on the floor, as there is a tendency to lift the heel slightly off the floor, which diminishes the stretch. Also, when you are stretching too hard, your knee may be bent slightly, decreasing the effectiveness of the stretch. The gastroc muscle connected to the Achilles tendon is tough and strong, so it's a good idea to hold this stretch for a longer period of time, leaning more toward the two-minute mark rather than just one minute.

## IT Band Stretch

I have a confession to make: I left this exercise for last because I rarely do this stretch as much as I do the others. Being that this area tends to be tight, you might wonder why.

This is a special area. Some people might think that the IT band is a muscle that you can stretch out, but it is a band that has many muscles connecting to it. The IT band is not a muscle itself, but a band made of other muscles. The two big muscles that connect at the top part of the IT band are the gluteus maximus (GM) and tensor fascia latae (TFL) muscle. The bottom part of the IT band connects into the tibialis anterior (TA) and the peroneus longus (PL). Therefore, there's a connection between the TFL and the TA, and another connection between the GM and PL. All of these muscles insert into one band. Therefore, trying to stretch the band instead of the muscles won't give you the stretch that you need. You won't elongate the band. More on that and foam rolling a little later.

Sometimes, this area tightens up because there's a muscle imbalance among the other muscles around the band. In my opinion, the best way to loosen the IT band and keep it loose is to strengthen the muscles around it, specifically the TFL, TA, the adductor muscles on the inner part of the thigh, and the gluteus medius muscle. This keeps the band taut and the leg balanced without the unnecessary pain and discomfort of foam rolling on the band. (Foam rolling is discussed in further detail in chapter 5.)

## EARLY STRENGTHENING EXERCISES

### Isometric Quad Contractions

Isometric exercises are great for when you want to do some sort of exercise, but you don't have much strength in the knee area. Research has shown that isometric exercise produces much less soreness the following day—sometimes, almost none at all.

Lie on the floor on your back. Place a towel underneath the back of your leg. Keep the noninjured leg bent in order to decrease pressure on your lower back. With your injured leg, try to push into the towel, thereby contracting your quadriceps muscle. You should maintain that contraction for five to ten seconds each time you perform the exercise.

*Your goal*: three sets of ten reps, holding for five to ten seconds, resting for thirty seconds in between each set.

**Isometric Quads in Prone**

This exercise strengthens the quads at the front of the thigh, and it is done this way to avoid back discomfort. Lie on your front with a rolled-up towel under the ankle, so the knee is slightly bent. Then push down on the towel, attempting to straighten the leg and contract the quads. Hold the position for five to ten seconds.

*Your goal*: three sets of ten reps, holding for five to ten seconds, resting for 30 seconds in between each set.

*What to watch out for*: Ensure that your ankle makes good contact with the towel and that your leg isn't raising off the ground with minimal contact. You should be pushing into the towel as hard as you can without hurting yourself.

**Isometric Hamstring Contractions**

This is a great exercise to strengthen your hamstrings and to balance them with your quadriceps.

Lie on your stomach and bend your injured knee. Have your partner or therapist hold your leg in a bent position, and when you are both ready, try bending your knee while your partner holds on to the back of your ankle, trying to prevent you from bending the knee. Hold that position for five to ten seconds, and then change the angle of your knee and do it again for ten repetitions.

*Your goal*: three sets of ten reps, holding for five to ten seconds, resting for thirty seconds in between each set.

*What to watch out for*: It's possible to do this exercise without a partner by placing the ankle of the noninjured leg behind the injured ankle to keep your injured leg from bending. You would then feel the isometric contraction in your hamstrings without actually moving your leg. It might be more difficult to do it by yourself then when someone is holding your leg for you, so pick the best option for you.

**Isometric Adductor Contraction**

The adductor muscle is often neglected when it comes to strengthening, and it therefore tends to be weak in people who have knee issues. Here's a great way to start getting them to contract.

Find a ball—I prefer a basketball or a soccer ball—and place it between your legs at the knees or just above your knees between your thighs. If you do not have a ball, roll up some bath or beach towels thickly enough that you can get a good squeeze from them. You can do this exercise either in a sitting position or by lying down with your knees bent; it's up to you. Squeeze the ball between your legs and hold the position for five to ten seconds each time.

*Your goal*: three sets of ten reps, holding for five to ten seconds, resting for thirty seconds in between each set.

## ISOTONIC KNEE EXERCISES

### Concentration Short Arc

This is an easy exercise to do that strengthens the muscles around your knee, specifically the part of your vastus medialis muscle that gets more attention from physiotherapists than any other part of a muscle, the vastus medialis oblique (VMO). The VMO is the section of the vastus medialis that is connected to your patella, and when it gets strong, it pulls the patella back into alignment and helps with proper tracking, which decreases cracking or other noises that you might hear.

Sit on the floor with your back straight and your arms off to your sides for support. Keep your unaffected leg bent at a 90-degree angle with your foot placed flat on the floor. Extend your injured leg straight out in front of you with your toes pointing toward the ceiling and the heel of your foot in contact with the floor. Put a small, rolled-up towel behind your injured knee.

While looking at your VMO—the inner part of your leg next to your kneecap—contract your quadriceps muscle, lifting your lower leg and heel off the ground and into the air in a slow and controlled motion. Make sure your ankle remains at a 90-degree angle, with your toes pointed toward the ceiling. Extend your lower leg as straight as possible without pain. Concentrate on holding the contraction for five seconds, and then slowly relax the muscle, allowing your lower leg to return to the ground. Relax the muscle and rest for five to ten seconds, and then repeat ten times.

*Your goal*: three sets of ten reps, holding for five to ten seconds, resting for thirty seconds in between reps.

*What to watch out for*: Make sure that you do this exercise within a pain-free range of motion only. If you feel pain or discomfort, try switching to a smaller towel or a small pillow to reduce stress and make your knee feel better. Do not continue this exercise if there is pain or swelling, and don't overdo it. My goals should act as a guideline for you. Everyone is different, and we must modify our activities based on what our body tells us. If you feel your muscles getting fatigued (a good thing) and you begin losing control (your leg begins twitching), stop and return to the exercise at another time. Do not perform this exercise on a soft surface (i.e., a bed), because you won't get the contraction that you want. Use smooth movements with this exercise and you will get a good contraction.

## Straight Leg Raise

This is a very popular exercise in our clinic. Also called a lock-and-lift exercise, it gets the quad muscle working.

Lying on your back, bend your noninjured leg approximately 90 degrees to protect your back from strain and place your foot flat on the floor. Tighten your quads, and lift your injured leg to the height of your bent knee quickly. It should take about one second. Hold the position for a couple of seconds, then slowly lower your leg. Control the descent of your leg, bringing it down to the floor in two to three seconds, always keeping the toes pointed upward.

*Your goal*: three sets of ten repetitions, resting for thirty seconds in between sets.

*What to watch out for*: Do not perform this exercise if your doctor or therapist believes that you have a disc herniation in your lower back. If you do, you might feel discomfort and pain every time you lift your leg. In fact, this exercise is a test for lower back pain that therapists might do, so get it cleared first from your therapist.

Another thing to look out for is your ability to keep your leg straight. If you can't keep the leg locked due to pain, you might have a strain or even a tear of your patellar tendon. In most cases, however, if the exercise is difficult without causing pain, you can continue practicing.

## Alphabet on Back

This is an exercise that I use to build the endurance of a muscle. This is essential for runners, cyclists, or just about anyone who doesn't want his or her leg to fatigue quickly but instead to stay strong throughout the day. Although the exercise is easy to understand, it is a challenge to finish on the first try.

Lying on your back, contract your quad muscle and lift your leg approximately 45 degrees. Then, using your leg, "write" the letters of the alphabet, from A to Z, using lowercase letters. Try to complete the entire alphabet without putting your foot down.

*Your goal*: one set of the alphabet from A through Z daily.

*What to watch out for*: Although this exercise might seem easy, people are surprised to find that's not always the case. You are moving your leg in the air throughout each letter of the alphabet without taking a break or stopping. If you must take a break because your leg is burning or you are tired, then please do so. Put your leg down, catch your breath, and when you are ready, continue from where you left off until you finish the alphabet. If your muscle isn't used to such endurance training, you'll feel a strong muscular burn. Do not arch your back when performing this exercise.

### Inside Straight Leg Raise

This exercise is basically the same as the straight leg raise, but it is performed on your side rather than your back. This really works the inside part of your leg, or your adductors, teaching them contract together with the rest of your leg muscles.

Lie on the side that your injured leg is on, bending the top leg and placing the foot of your top leg on the floor behind the injured leg. Make sure that you are fully leaning on your side and are not half-turned on your back. Point your toes toward your head and lift your leg toward the ceiling quickly, in about a second, and then slowly lower the leg with control all the way down. It should take two to three seconds.

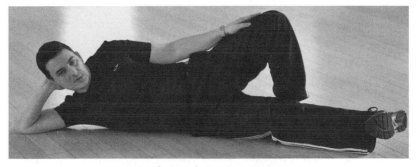

Inside Straight Leg Raise Begin.

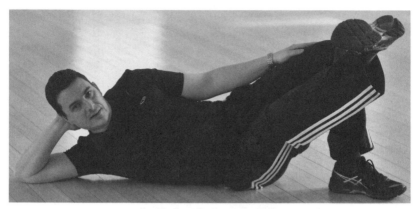

Inside Straight Leg Raise End.

*Your goal*: three sets of ten reps, resting for thirty seconds in between sets.

*What to watch out for*: The tendency to lean back rather than to stay strictly on your side changes the exercise from an inside straight leg raise to a standard straight leg raise. When performing this exercise, it is typical to feel a burn either at the top of the muscle near the pelvic or groin area, in the middle of the muscle, or sometimes even at the joint area of the knee. It is also normal for the opposite leg, especially the hamstring, to contract hard or, in some rare cases, to spasm. This may be due to the fact that you need to contract or push with your noninjured leg in order to lift your injured leg off the ground. If this happens to you, don't get discouraged. It is normal, and you'll improve with consistent practice. Once the exercise becomes easy, add a one-pound ankle weight, eventually moving up to a five-pound weight. Once you have attained that level, you can move onto another exercise altogether.

### Inside Alphabet

This exercise is basically the previous alphabet exercise, but it is performed on your side. Fair warning: you'll really feel your muscles working during this exercise, and you may experience muscle burn in a way you've never felt before.

Lie on the side that your injured leg is on, bending the top leg and placing the foot of your top leg on the floor behind the injured leg. Make sure that you are fully leaning on your side and are not half-turned on your back. Then, using your leg, "write" the letters of the alphabet, from A to Z, using lowercase letters. Try to complete the entire alphabet without putting your foot down.

*Your goal*: one set of the alphabet from A through Z daily.

*What to watch out for*: Make sure that you are lying on your side while performing this exercise. Again, it is OK to stop if you have to. Catch your breath and continue. Eventually, you'll become a pro and finish the whole alphabet without stopping. When that movement becomes too easy, start using ankle weights. Begin with a very light weight, say one pound, and work your way up to a five-pound weight. When you can perform the movement using that weight comfortably, you can stop this exercise.

## The Bridge

This is an exercise that most people neglect. The gluteus maximus and gluteus medius help to stabilize the knee, not allowing it to collapse. If you sit in a chair all day, your glutes flatten out and become weaker and weaker. This is great for strengthening those muscles, creating a better balance of strength between the front and back. The bridge is also important for improving core stabilization while the hips are extending. This is very important in protecting your lower back from pain and discomfort, because your lower back must be stabilized during lower body extension to reduce strain on your spine.

Start by lying faceup on the floor with arms to the sides, knees bent at 90 degrees. Keep your heels flat on the ground. Tighten your abs. Lift your hips off the ground until your knees, hips, and shoulders are in a

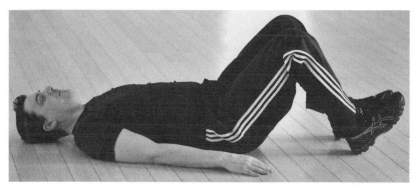

Bridging Begin.

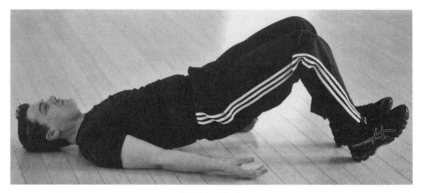

Bridging End.

straight line, making sure to squeeze your glutes as you reach the top of the movement. Also, imagine that your knees are moving away from you as you keep your abs tight. Your weight should be balanced between your shoulders and your feet. Hold for two to three seconds at the top of the movement, then slowly lower your hips back to the ground, allowing them to slightly touch the ground before completing another rep.

*Your goal*: three sets of ten repetitions, holding for thirty seconds in between sets.

*What to watch out for*: There are different variations of this exercise that you can try. If you are able, try it with only the heels of your feet and shoulders touching the floor. This is more difficult because your heel provides less stability than the entire foot. You'll feel it more in your hamstring region. Also, if you're feeling a pull on your quads, that's a good thing. You're stretching your quads as you're contracting your glutes and hamstrings, so in effect, you're starting to balance out your leg strength, making it equal in every direction.

Eventually, you can move to one leg on the floor with the other leg straight in the air or cross your good leg over the top of your bad leg.

### Clamshells

As I've said before, strengthening your glute muscles, especially your gluteus medius, is very important for proper knee control and for preventing it from bending inward when squatting down. The gluteus medius pulls your leg to the outside, which keeps your leg aligned when bending or squatting down. Therefore the muscles that externally rotate the hips are an important area to strengthen.

Lie on the floor on your side. Bend your knees slightly, keeping your body straight. Put your hand on your hip to help you stay straight and not rotate your body (thus working your lower back rather than the hip area). You can feel your glute muscle working when you leave your hand there.

Keeping both of your knees bent, bring the top knee upward, as if you are the top shell of a clam opening up. Hold that position for two to three seconds and slowly return to the starting position.

*Your goal*: three sets of ten repetitions, holding for two to three seconds, resting for thirty seconds in between each set.

*What to watch out for*: This exercise is done mostly with the knees bent, making it a little easier because the hip flexors are involved. If you do it with your thighs straight, it stretches the hip flexors and works the gluteus medius region, providing a much stronger contraction. It also makes the exercise much harder than the original version. An elastic resistance band around your legs also provides a good burn. This exercise should be a challenge, but, above all, you should be able to feel the appropriate area working. That should always be the goal of every exercise.

## Side-Lying Hip Abduction

This is by far my favorite exercise to suggest to patients for strengthening their gluteus medius muscle. Apart from being easy to understand and perform, it has been shown that this exercise is the most effective in stimulating the gluteus medius.

Lying on your side, keeping your hips in a neutral position, turn your leg inward so that your toes point down and your heel points up. Lift your leg all the way up quickly, about one second, then slowly lower it down, keeping it turned inward throughout the movement.

*Your goal*: three sets of ten repetitions, resting for thirty seconds in between sets.

*What to watch for*: You can obviously perform the exercise with the leg in a neutral position (knees straight instead of pointing down). However, I've found that you can get a better contraction with your leg pointing downward, contracting an already stretched muscle. Try it both ways and see what works for you. Work up to five pounds using ankle weights.

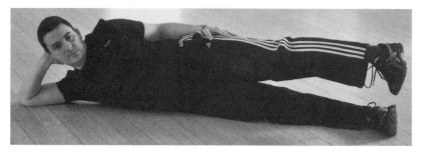

Side-Lying Hip Abduction Begin.

### Side-Lying Hip Circles

This is the same position as the side-lying hip abduction exercise, but instead of lifting your leg up and down, you move your leg in circles.

Keeping your toes pointing down and the leg up, make large circles ten times, going in one direction. Then perform ten circles moving in the opposite direction.

*Your goal*: three sets of ten repetitions, breaking for thirty seconds in between each set.

*What to watch out for*: Moving your leg in one direction is typically more difficult than moving it the other direction. Most people find that it's much tougher to swing the leg backward than it is to swing it forward.

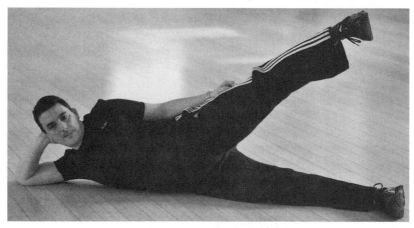

Side-Lying Hip Abduction End.

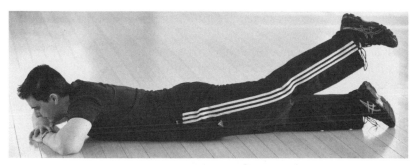

Prone Hip Raise Knee Bending Begin.

That's to be expected, since your hip flexors usually are stronger than your glute muscles. Keep working it in both directions, again working up to five pounds using ankle weights. Be sure to balance on your hips without falling too far forward or backward.

**Prone Hip Raise Knee Bending**

Along with the bridge, this is a great starter exercise to strengthen the hamstrings and the glute region. It is easy to do, and you'll get great results.

Lying on your stomach, lift your injured leg into the air, just enough to clear the quadriceps off the floor. Bend and straighten your knee for a series of ten repetitions while the leg remains in the air.

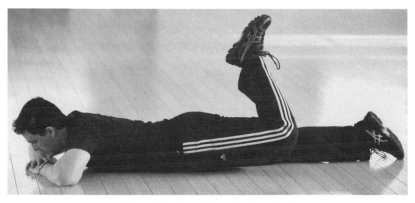

Prone Hip Raise Knee Bending End.

*Your goal*: three sets of ten repetitions, resting for thirty seconds in between sets.

*What to watch out for*: Don't lift your leg too high—it should just clear the floor—otherwise you risk placing a rotational strain on your lower back.

### Prone Hip Raise Circles

This is the same position as the side-lying hip circles exercises above, but this time you'll be making big circles going in both directions.

*Your goal*: three sets of ten reps in each direction, resting for thirty seconds in between reps.

*What to watch out for*: Again, avoid lifting your leg too high, causing back strain. You should feel muscle burn primarily in the glutes region and upper hamstrings. Take a short break between reps and switch directions, circling the other way. One last thing: Don't worry if your circles aren't perfect—no one will know! The circular motion is what's important.

### Wall Sits

Wall sits, sometimes called wall squats, are great for building strength in your quad muscles, as well as for stabilizing contractions in your glutes and upper hamstring muscles. This exercise greatly helps people who suffer from runner's knee or patellar tendinitis.

Standing against a wall, move your feet about two feet in front of the wall. Your legs should be about shoulder width apart.

Slowly bend your knees and slide down the wall until your thighs are parallel to the floor or until your knees are at 90-degree angles. Make sure that your knee joints are aligned over your ankle joints, in which case you may need to inch your feet further from the wall. Hold the position for about fifteen to thirty seconds, working your way to a sixty-second hold.

*Your goal*: three sets of ten reps, holding for fifteen to thirty seconds (but working toward sixty seconds), breaking for thirty seconds in between sets.

*What to watch out for*: Make sure your shins are parallel to the wall, and don't let your knees extend past your toes. Also, try not to allow your shoulders to slump forward. Keep your back straight the whole time.

To slide down the wall more easily, place a Swiss ball or gym ball behind your lower back. To make it more challenging, take one foot off the floor and then put it back down after a few seconds. To work your calves at the same time, alternate between lifting your left heel for a few seconds and then your right.

Once you get the hang of this exercise and it starts to become easy, you can start with weights in your hands.

## Step Ups

Another great exercise for strengthening your glutes, upper hamstrings, and knee are step ups.

Before starting this exercise, find a chair or bench to place your foot on so that your knee bends at a 90-degree angle. Weight benches are often the ideal height, but your dining room chairs may also be the appropriate size for this exercise.

Start by placing your entire right foot onto the bench or chair. Press your weight through your right heel as you step onto the bench, bringing your left foot next to your right so that you are standing with both feet on the bench. Then, return to the starting position by stepping down with the right foot then the left so that both feet are on the floor.

Try to do about ten to fifteen steps leading with the left foot, then repeat another ten to fifteen steps with your right foot. This may feel tough at first, but if you keep at it, your legs will get stronger and you will become more comfortable.

*Your goal*: three sets of ten to fifteen reps for each leg, breaking for thirty seconds in between sets.

## Side Plank Isometric Abduction

Although this might at first seem an odd choice, I believe that the oblique muscles play a vital role in stabilizing your pelvis and keeping everything in place. If you are a runner, this exercise should become part of your workout routine.

Lie on the floor on your right side with your legs extended and your feet and hips resting on the ground on top of each other. Place your right elbow directly under your shoulder to prop up your torso, and align your head with your spine. Gently contract your core and lift your hips and knees off the floor. Hold for ten to thirty seconds, gradually working up to a minute, and return to the starting position. Roll onto the other side and repeat.

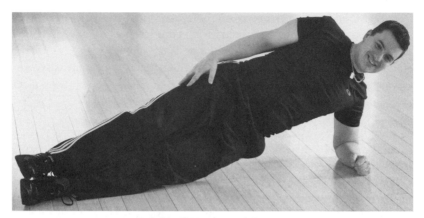

Side Plank Isometric Abduction.

*Your goal*: three sets of ten reps, holding for thirty seconds (gradually increasing to sixty seconds), resting for thirty seconds in between sets.

*What to watch out for*: Make sure that you are lifting from your pelvis and not pushing from your shoulder. Try to feel it on the sides of your abs. Also, keep your head facing straight ahead, not looking toward your knees. If the exercise is too hard to begin with, start with bent knees rather than straight. It decreases leverage and makes the exercise slightly easier. When holding this position becomes too easy, you can progress to moving up and down for three sets of twenty reps.

### The Stork

As stated earlier, balance and proprioception are important components of knee injury rehabilitation. Good balance makes your knee, hip, and ankle work together in unison.

Begin by standing on your injured leg with your eyes open for thirty seconds. It might sound easy, but if your leg is wobbling and you are struggling to maintain your balance, your leg might not be as strong as you think. Keep working at it until you maintain straight posture and are in control of your balance. When thirty seconds seems easy, increase to sixty seconds.

When you feel comfortable and strong on your leg with your eyes open, it's time to move to the next phase: standing on one leg with your eyes closed. For obvious reasons, please have a chair, desk, or something to hold on to in case you lose your balance. Many people are surprised about the degree of difficulty of this exercise when you close your eyes. The main difference is that when your eyes are open, you can adjust your body with visual clues. When your eyes are closed, your body has to rely on other senses; in this case, kinesthetic sense, which we all have, though we don't use it enough. Again, try to hold your position without falling or hopping around for thirty seconds. Eventually work up to a sixty-second hold.

*Your goal*: three reps of thirty seconds on each leg with eyes open, breaking for ten to fifteen seconds in between reps. Repeat with your eyes closed.

*What to watch out for*: Please don't fall. It takes time and practice to master this exercise, but it makes your leg work more efficiently. Eventually, you can progress to uneven surfaces, like a wobble board, a bosu ball, or any device that isn't fully stable when you stand on it. Again, please do these exercises near something sturdy, should you need to balance yourself.

Please know that this is not a complete list of every knee rehabilitation exercise out there. There are many others using different methods and techniques. You can do some exercises with free weights, elastic bands, tubes, canes, hockey sticks, or even water bottles! The most important thing is the result: Does the exercise give you what you need? Do you feel it in the area that you are supposed to?

## KNEE ROUTINES

What follow are some examples of routines that I know will be helpful in strengthening your leg and reducing the pain in your knees. However, please note that these are generalized programs. If your doctor or therapist has prescribed a specific program of exercises, you should follow it instead. Please consult with your health professional if you have questions or concerns about any of these routines.

### Level 1 Exercises

1. Heel to behind 3 × 10
2. Prolonged knee extension 3 × 1-minute hold
3. Prolonged knee flexion 3 × 1-minute hold

4. Hip internal rotation self-stretching 3 × 1-minute hold
5. Isometric quad contractions 3 × 10 with 5–10-second hold
6. Isometric hamstring contractions 3 × 10 with 5–10-second hold
7. Isometric adductor contraction 3 × 10 with  5–10-second hold

**Level 2 Exercises**

1. Quadriceps stretch 3 × 1-minute hold
2. Hamstring stretch 3 × 1-minute hold
3. Concentration short arc 3 × 10
4. Straight leg raise 3 × 10
5. Alphabet on back × 1
6. Inside straight leg raise 3 × 10
7. Inside alphabet × 1

**Level 3 Exercises**

1. Clamshells 3 × 10
2. Side-lying hip abduction 3 × 10
3. Side-lying hip circles 3 × 10, both directions
4. Bridge 3 × 10 both legs, eventually moving to one leg
5. Prone hip raise knee bending 3 × 10
6. Prone hip circles 3 × 10, both directions

**Level 4 Exercises**

1. Wall sits 3 × 10 with 15–30-second hold
2. Side plank isometric abdominal 3 × 30 seconds
3. Step ups 3 × 10
4. The stork 3 × 30 seconds eyes open, 3 × 30 seconds eyes closed

## SUMMARY

- A twenty-minute warm up prepares your heart, nervous system, and muscles to work out and hedges against injury.
- Stretching is recommended every day for best results. If you miss a day, that's OK as long as you resume the following day. Consistency with stretching is much more important than the intensity of the stretch.

- The eccentric phase of an exercise repetition is just as important as if not more important than the concentric phase of a movement. Therefore, it should be given equal attention in order to achieve the kind of balance that prevents injuries.
- The 3x10 exercise routine formula—three sets of ten repetitions—increases the endurance and strength of muscles effectively and safely.
- Working the glutes, especially the gluteus medius, helps to stabilize the pelvis and reduces pressure on the knee. It is a vital part of any knee program.
- Working on balance and proprioception, an often-forgotten element of rehab programs, helps the muscles work in unison. When the knee, hip, and ankle contract and work together, movements both in sports and everyday living are that much easier.

# 5

# Running

Running is the greatest metaphor for life, because you get out of it what you put into it.

—Oprah Winfrey

Running is no big deal when you think about it. It's basically putting one foot in front of the other. For millions of people, it's an extremely enjoyable way of working out. You could call it the best type of cardio training out there. According to the American College of Cardiology, running at slow speeds (I think of it as slow jogging) can reduce the risk of dying from a cardiac or cardiovascular disease.

Why do people like it so much? I'm sure you've heard people explain that running is like a drug and they have to keep doing it. They're kind of right. When you run, your brain pumps out two powerful feel-good chemicals, endorphins and endocannabinoids. Does that last word sound like a real drug? There's a reason. Chemically, the endocannabinoids your body produces during a run aren't all that different from marijuana's mood-altering chemical, THC. During about the midpoint of your run, your body releases a special kind of endocannabinoids called anandamide, and that's the state that runners refer to as the "runner's high."

A *Medicine and Science in Sports and Exercise* study of nearly 100,000 runners and walkers found that, believe it or not, running doesn't increase the risk of osteoarthritis—even people who cover 26.2 miles on a regular basis. In fact, the study showed that runners were half as likely to suffer from knee osteoarthritis compared with walkers. It seems like the opposite should be true, but here's why. Every time you pound the pavement, you stress your bones and cartilage, just like your muscles, causing

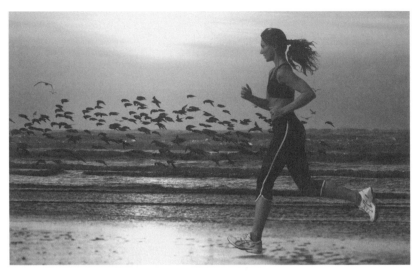

Running on Beach. *EnjoyLife, image from Bigstockphoto.com*

them to spring back stronger. Low-impact exercises like walking, or even spinning or swimming, don't offer this bone-building benefit. So when people who obviously don't run tell you that running can be bad for you, tell them about this study.

The most common knee injury among runners is the one aptly called "runner's knee" or patellofemoral pain syndrome (PFPS), which was discussed in previous chapters. This is the most common overuse injury among runners. Tight hamstring and calf muscles put pressure on the knee, and weak quadriceps and gluteal muscles can cause the patella to track out of alignment. This is sometimes due to iliotibial band (ITB) syndrome. The IT band itself becomes irritated due to continual compression on the outside of your knee, causing an irritation or swelling of the fat pad between the bone and the tendon on the side of the knee. ITB syndrome can also be caused by poor physical condition, not warming up before exercise, or drastic changes in activity levels.

The problem is with how the IT band functions with the rest of the body when we run. The IT band is a thick, wide, hard band that extends from the tensor fascia lata muscle and the glute muscles, which are found on the outside part of your leg and knee. It connects to the lateral part of the femur bone to an area called the lateral condyle. This is simple but significant: the IT band does not contract. Its function is to stabilize the knee when fully extended and partially flexed, which happens during running. It is a band of dense fiber, not a muscle itself. There are the muscles around it that contract the band, including the tensor fascia lata (TFL) muscle and the glutes.

To decrease stress and pain in your knees, try modifying your running. For example, some people can't run on hills because the inclination puts additional pressure on the knees and causes problems. Cross-training can be a good option until the pain subsides, but cyclists also frequently struggle with IT band problems from the repetitive motion of pedaling. A popular technique that many people use is foam rolling on the IT band itself.

Foam rolling is a self-myofascial release (SMR) technique used by athletes and physical therapists to aid with muscle recovery. Fascia, the soft tissue portion of the connective tissue in the muscle that provides support and protection, can become restricted due to overuse, trauma, and inactivity. Consequently, inflammation occurs, and if it becomes bad enough, the connective tissue can thicken, which results in pain, irritation, and additional inflammation. Although religiously rolling out your IT band might feel good, the idea that you are going to relax or release the IT band is incorrect. The phrase "rolling out your IT band" itself makes it sound like you are rolling out a piece of dough, but your IT band is anything but pliable. It's a remarkably strong piece of connective tissue, and research has shown that it cannot be released or manipulated by manual techniques such as foam rolling. If you try to smooth out areas of inflammation, you'll only increase inflammation. That's why you are in pain so much. And if you are in pain, your body will be too stressed to repair itself. I personally never recommend foam rolling the IT band. You are not helping yourself. Continually trying to foam roll the IT band not only fails to work, but it irritates the fat pad located at the knee, as well as compresses the vastus lateralis muscle. Soft tissue release should be done at the TFL and gluteus medius muscles, both of which directly place tension to the fascia but play no role in the "release" of the fascial band itself, which is stuck by fascia to the femur along its length.

Multiple studies have found that one of the leading causes of ITB syndrome is weakness in the hip and glute muscles, which then pull on the IT band.[1] Some of the exercises that were explained in chapter 4 for the glute area like clamshells, side-lying abductions and circles, and bridging can be much more helpful. These exercises are not just rehab but can help prevent problems in the first place.

It's also common for mechanical issues to contribute to IT band stress. Overpronating or supinating as you land can stress the IT band. When fatigue sets in, many runners tend to collapse their ankles or knees inward, which then pulls on the band running along the outside of the leg.

So what is overpronation? It is a term that runners talk about frequently and a problem for many people. Let's start with pronation first. Pronation is the way your foot rolls inward when you walk and run. This happens so that your leg can absorb the impact and shock from everyday walking and running. The outside part of the heel makes initial contact, and as the force gets transmitted forward, the ankle starts to roll in. The normal level of rolling in or pronating is about fifteen degrees or so. Everyone has to pronate. However, some people tend to roll inward a little more, or overpronate, whereas others roll in less than the norm, or underpronate. Most people who come to the physiotherapy clinic for running problems tend to overpronate. This means the foot and ankle have problems stabilizing the body, and shock isn't absorbed as efficiently. At the end of the walking cycle, called your gait, the front of the foot pushes off the ground using mainly the big toe and second toe, which then must do all the work. Overpronation can stress and tighten your muscles, so do a little extra stretching. Too much motion of the foot can cause issues with your ankle and place undue stress to your knee and hip.

Good, hard orthotics can help hold up the inside arch of your foot, called the medial arch. If the arch is held up and maintained, overpronation is minimized. Although that's true and orthotics are ideal for some really bad arch conditions, there are some other alternatives.

The main one is strengthening specific muscles from your abs all the way down to your feet. When your foot overpronates, the following happens at the other joints: Your knee and hip joint internally rotate or turn inward and your knee bends inward, moving toward your other knee. Your pelvis turns forward, toward the ground instead of staying straight up. All of these excessive, unbalanced motions place stress on your joints. Eventually, through the wear and tear of everyday walking, you might develop osteoarthritis of your knee, which causes significant pain and stiffness.

A lot of lower limb problems can be successfully treated by your doctor, physical therapist or allied health professional. Everybody is unique and special, and every person has subtle differences in their bodies that must be assessed. What I am offering is a guide to helping you understand what is happening and some things that you can do with the help of your therapist.

Strengthening your glute muscles, especially your gluteus medius muscle, has been shown to help with stability of the pelvis and, combined with your gluteus maximus training, can help keep your pelvis in the proper position and take some stress off your knee.[2] In addition, strengthening the adductor muscles on the inner part of the thigh balances out the strength in the knee, bringing the kneecap to the center rather than off to the side, thereby decreasing the imbalances and strengthening the leg. It is also important to maintain a flexibility routine for your quads, hams, hips, and glutes muscles to keep them flexible and loose.

In the ankle region, strengthening your tibialis posterior muscle is helpful. When running, the tibialis posterior slows down the movement of active pronation from heel strike to toe off. So for those of us who overpronate or pronate very rapidly, our tibialis posterior muscle has to work hard to help control this movement. If it is weak, it can't slow down the pronation, allowing the overpronation to happen.

What about the little muscles in your foot? Do they play a role in helping with controlling your pronation movement? Your foot has approximately four layers of muscles that control movements in your foot, which are called intrinsic foot muscles, or IFM for short. Research has shown that the IFM muscles play a critical role in stabilizing the foot mechanics when you are standing on one leg. They also provide support to your arch when you are walking, as well as being responsible for keeping the shape of the arch on the inside of your foot.

Another way to help decrease your foot pronation and also to reduce the need for expensive orthotics is to train another muscle in your foot called the abductor hallucis muscle. The abductor hallucis muscle plays an important role in maintaining arch height of the inner part of your foot, as well as controlling overpronation. This muscle flexes and abducts your big toe, prevents overrotation of your tibia, and decreases the inversion, or turning in, of your heel bone, called the calcaneus. Strengthening this muscle can aid in supporting your arch and preventing excessive pronation, which will decrease some of your running injuries.

So what kind of exercises can you do to strengthen these little muscles and to help with the arch of the foot? Here are some examples:

*Bunching up a towel with your toes*: Keeping your foot flat, try curling in your toes and hold the position between three and five seconds and then let go. Focus on squeezing your toes as much as you can. This is an exercise that you can do anywhere.

*Picking up marbles or other small objects with your feet*: This is essentially the same concept but a little more fun. It forces your muscles to hold the marble while moving your foot to put them in a different place.

*Pointing at objects around the room with your foot*: This offers the benefit of strengthening your foot muscles in all the different directions and making your muscles work in new and different ways.

*Separating your toes and then squishing them together*: This is probably one of the hardest and sometimes most unusual movements to do, because your muscles are not used to moving that way. This exercise wakes up these muscles and rids them of their "amnesia."

*Walking on sand*: If you have access to a beach, walking on the sand is one of the best exercises you can do to strengthen the foot. Because your foot sinks in, the sand provides resistance and makes your muscles work in different ways than they are accustomed to.

Like every other muscle in the body, building strength takes time. Be consistent with exercising the intrinsic muscles and you'll reap the benefits of a strong foot.

Keep in mind that a combination of strengthening the muscles in the feet along with the muscles along the leg all the way to the gluteus medius muscles and abdominals will help you to maintain the balance and support in your leg, reduce any stresses in your knee and other joints, and help improve your running.

The position that your foot ideally should be in is a neutral position. That position is when your feet are pointed straight ahead, not turned out, and are parallel to each other. Your muscles—and your entire system—are designed to be their strongest and most secure in this position.

Sitting on the couch binge watching your favorite TV show might be relaxing, but doing so on a daily basis is not good for your body. If you are always sitting—whether working at your desk or surfing on your laptop—your muscles and joints start to atrophy because they are not being used or stimulated. Forward head, rolled-in shoulders, and a hunched posture weakens your body. Sitting also weakens all the muscles around your hips, especially your glute muscles. When the glutes get weak, your power also weakens, because your hips generate most of your power, whether it is in running outside, playing your favorite sport, or bending over to pick something up from the floor. Not using your foot muscles can also weaken them.

What can we do to remedy this? We buy shoes that provide a lot of support and cost $150! In some cases, people use orthotic shoe inserts for additional support. It's like running with a cast on! I think that one of the issues that runners generally have is weak feet. We train the other parts of our body until we can't push ourselves anymore, but the shoe that we use is so strong that it results in the same deleterious effects that sitting has on our glutes. It's been estimated that close to $6 billion is spent on running shoes on an annual basis. There are three main types of running shoes marketed today: the stability shoe, the motion-control shoe, and the minimalistic shoe. Most times, a running shoe store or sports clinic will watch the way that you run and will put you in the correct type of shoe, depending on how much you pronate.

If you are a slight to moderate pronator, then you are a good candidate for a stability shoe. If you are flat-footed and a severe pronator, then you are placed with a motion-control shoe with tons of padding everywhere, which is like wearing a rigid boot.

You might be thinking that significant research goes into shoe design. Unfortunately, it is the science of marketing by the big corporations rather than any valid scientific research that specific shoes prevent injury. Yes, you read correctly. There is no real scientific research behind the fact that a specific shoe helps runners perform better than any other shoe. There is also no research that you should buy a spanking new pair of shoes after every 500 miles—or that it will keep you healthier and decrease the number of foot and knee injuries. If that was the case, runners would never have any injuries due to running; yet in clinics across the country, there are many, from the novice to the professional, with running-related injuries. The best way to help yourself avoid running-related injuries is to achieve neutral foot position. Well, in that case, what about the minimalistic shoe? Yes, it offers less support, but it is still costly and sometimes causes even greater problems than before. Why is that? People are always looking for a quick fix, but if you abruptly switched from a stability or motion-controlled shoe to a minimal shoe, your muscles and ligaments can't handle this newfound stress when you are pounding on the pavement. This is when your Achilles tendon gets inflamed and you develop shin splints or other reasons to visit your friendly neighborhood physical therapist or allied health professional.

If you look at people from different cultures around the world that go barefoot, you'll notice that they have strong, equally balanced foot muscle strength with good arches. You've heard stories about young kids in these countries who can run for a long time without shoes and without injuries. It's been shown that the runners in Ancient Greece ran barefoot.

In Christopher McDougall's popular book *Born to Run*, the author writes about the Tarahumara Indians in Mexico's Copper Canyon who are able to run pain free and without injury for hundreds of miles. The Tarahumara Indians can run this way into their seventies with no issues. It is surprising to most people that this is possible.

Research studies have demonstrated some interesting facts. It has been found that when people run wearing running shoes, they tend to land on their heels, making use of the pad that's built into the shoes. Landing this way sends a massive jolt of force upward through your ankles, knees, hips, and into your spine. However, when runners were evaluated running barefoot, they tended to land through their forefoot or midfoot, with the landing point nearer to the body's center of mass, where you want the force to be, not outward toward the front of the body.

Barefoot runners use the natural shock-absorbing, spring-like mechanism of the muscles, ligaments, and tendons within and around the foot, ankle, knee, and hip.

What about the people who have lived for thousands of years without extensively padded shoes or without anything more than sandals? Runners ran successfully until the 1970s with shoes that had no padding, no pronation or stability control, no expensive orthotics, and no high-tech materials.

I'm not suggesting that we should toss our running shoes into the garbage, but rather that we should be aware of the research out there before buying that expensive new shoe with all the "extras" that the manufacturers claim will make your running that much better or smoother.

What about flip-flops? There are some cultures that wear them all the time. If you look at their feet, they tend to be flat-footed or have "island feet." Not a good idea, because it alters normal foot mechanics by changing the ability of your big toe to move properly. Flip-flops make your big toe contract or "clench" to hold on to the flip-flop when you are walking. This shortens the tissues in your arch, changing the mechanics and stress to your plantar fascia, which can create plantar fasciitis as well as a shortened Achilles tendon, causing tendinitis and pain.

If you really want to switch from your super-padded shoe to a minimalistic shoe, please do so slowly and gradually. If you make the change too quickly, it's too much change too fast on your legs, and you'll injure yourself. I implore you to start working on the weak muscles of your foot and getting your big toe and little muscles stronger. Definitely start working on your balance (without shoes) in eyes open and closed positions (please, have something next to you to hold on to if needed). Give the transition time: it might take a couple of months for your body to get accustomed to wearing your new shoes. Also start with short distances with your new shoes and gradually build up the distance—about a 10 percent boost each run. Keep the urge of running like the Flash to a minimum in the beginning. Above all, pick a pair of shoes that are comfortable and that you like. If you decide to invest in zero-drop shoes, please go slowly, especially if you started with a shoe with a twelve-millimeter drop with motion control for stability. Transitioning abruptly from a shoe with a fully cushioned heel to a no-heel shoe is asking for trouble. If you progress slowly and steadily and keep working on the power and strength of your feet, including your big toe, you'll see the difference and your running will improve greatly.

A small point about the way you walk: First, stand up and look at your feet. Are they facing forward or pointed outward? Some people have a tendency of walking with turn-out feet syndrome, or walking "like a duck." When you walk this way, your stability suffers, and with each step, it gets worse and worse. Your foot splays outward, the arches in your foot start to collapse, ankles and knees turn inward, and hips fall forward. These improper shearing forces start to rub on your joints, creating pain and discomfort. Also, when you walk with your feet turned out, your quad tendon is not perpendicular to your patella, but it has to be if you want to be perfectly aligned and not off-center. Think about such misalignment in relation to the number of steps that you take per hour, per day, et cetera, which may explain why you have patella tendinitis or an Achilles tendon problem.

## PROPER POSTURE HELPS YOUR RUNNING

Why would a proper neutral spine help? Running involves the lower body, not the upper, right? This does not seem to be the case. If your spine is in the proper position, your movements become more efficient. This means that your muscles require less energy to keep you straight, and more power and energy can be directed to your lower body.

Good posture means maintaining a neutral spine throughout your body. Having a neutral spine means achieving the three natural curves that keep your spine healthy, happy, and long lasting.

The three natural curves of the spine are the cervical, thoracic, and lumbar regions. You might also hear (especially Pilates fanatics) about a neutral pelvis. This means trying to get the top of your pelvic bone—your anterior superior iliac spine, commonly called your ASIS—in a vertical line with your pubic symphysis, which is an area made of cartilage that separates your left hip or pubic bone from your right hip.

When your therapist looks at your posture, he or she is looking to see if you deviate from the middle, or plumb, line. We look at you from the front, side, and back to see if your head is too far forward, if your shoulders turn in, if your pelvis is rotated, along with a host of other things. We examine you from your head down to your feet for anything that looks different from the norm.

It's important to know that proper posture should be maintained while sitting, standing, and sleeping. Why should we maintain good posture? Other than the obvious reason—avoiding injury—another reason is to try to keep the body's different parts in the proper position so that the least amount of energy is required to maintain a position that you want, placing the least amount of stress on the body's tissues. You will also receive a lot of positive looks coming your way, as people admire your amazing posture, whether standing or sitting, almost in the same way that people gawk at someone who is in shape and walks proudly because of it.

So what does it mean to have poor posture? What poor posture means is that your body has developed muscle imbalances due to your daily activities and habits. Some of your muscles shorten or tighten up, while other muscles stretch out and lengthen, providing no support at all. Repetitive movements and other biomechanical factors, such as different forces placed on your body, can create postural problems. It also has been shown that workers with higher stress levels are more prone to develop neck and shoulder symptoms.

Poor posture can contribute to chest pain. This is because of the hunched or slouched sitting position we use at our desks during the day. Your lungs can't fully expand and your shoulders turn inward, causing your pectoral muscles to tighten up. You start taking shallow breaths, and chest pain starts to develop. Large-breasted women develop this problem of hunching and rotating their shoulders inward.

It's rare to see someone with a strong upper and lower back and a very weak front. As humans, we tend to look at and train the areas of our body that we see on a daily basis. We normally look at the front of our body, and want to make it look better and stronger. We forget to look at our back part of our body, basically because we don't look at it as much. If we trained and took care of the back part of us as much as we do the front part, we would have fewer postural issues and definitely less pain and discomfort.

Most, but not all, posture-related problems result from sitting. As a society, we watch more television than any other previous generation. We drive and fly more now than in the past, often in poorly designed seats. A lot of us work sedentary jobs day after day or sit in front of computer terminals. Daily improper, repetitive positions can cause havoc with your body. Some other factors that can contribute to poor posture include excessive weight; a mattress or pillow that isn't right for you, causing poor sleep support; improper shoes; careless sitting or standing habits (I am guilty of this one as well); a poorly designed workspace; and, as stated before, occupational stress.

## FORWARD HEAD POSTURE

Did you know that your head on your spine weighs approximately twelve pounds? It's not uncommon for a patient to come into the clinic with a head that has moved from one to three inches forward from the shoulders. That's forty-two pounds that your posterior neck muscles have to hold up all day, every day! Eventually, these muscles throw in the towel and call it a day. The way they do that is by sending you a pain signal to stop you from holding that position.

When the head is that far forward—adding forty-two pounds of additional leverage and pull on the cervical spine (neck region)—it can pull the spine out of normal alignment. According to Dr. Rene Caillet, MD, a forward head posture can result in a loss of 30 percent of an individual's vital lung capacity due to the loss of the cervical lordosis (the natural curvature of the neck). By decreasing the cervical lordosis, this forward head posture limits the hyoid muscle's action to lift the first rib when inhaling. The gastrointestinal region, especially the large intestine, becomes irritated from the forward neck posture, which can cause sluggish bowel function and execution. This is a serious thing to consider. Dr. Caillet advises patients to work on the head position before working on the body, because the head is the first part to move and the body follows it.

So what kind of exercises can you do to give yourself a flexible and mobile thoracic spine?

## THORACIC SPINE WALL EXERCISE

This exercise does wonders for your rib cage area and can help straighten your spine. It looks easy, but please move into it slowly.

Place your back against the wall, with your lower back flat, causing the lower part of your pelvis to tilt forward. Lift both arms up to 90 degrees. Bend your arms. If at some point you feel pulling in your rib cage or thoracic spine movement, hold the position for five seconds and release. If it is not pulling in that position, bend your arms and try to place them against the wall. Most people feel the stretch at this point. If not, slowly slide your arms up, until you feel a pull in your spine.

*Your goal:* one set of five reps, holding for five seconds (when you are able to comfortably do so, gradually increase to ten repetitions, holding for ten seconds).

*What to watch out for:* Your lower back arching. Make sure it is flat against the wall. Also try to keep your head and arms against the wall when performing the exercise.

## AIRPLANE

This exercise will work on the muscles in your shoulder, upper back, and all the muscles in between. It strengthens your postural muscles and gives you that tall, erect look. The reason it is named the airplane is because if it is done properly, you will look like an airplane.

Lying on your stomach, bring your shoulder blades together and your head slightly back; turn your hands outward so that your thumbs point to the ceiling. Hold the position for ten seconds. Progress this exercise with hand weights of one pound in each hand, gradually increasing to five pounds.

*Your goal:* one set of ten repetitions, holding for ten seconds, resting for ten seconds between each rep.

*What to watch out for:* The way you are turning your arms. If you are performing the exercise correctly, you will be able to bring the shoulder blades really close together. If you turn your arms the other way, your shoulder blades will be further apart. Use the way when your shoulder blades are close together.

## SUPERMAN

This really works on bringing your shoulders back, opening you up, and making you look straight and tall again, instead of the hunched-over posture that most of us develop at work. It is one of the best scapular stabilizing exercises, and you can do it anywhere. It is called superman because you will look like you are flying.

Start by lying on your stomach, bringing your arms toward your head, shoulder width apart. Point your thumbs toward the ceiling. In this position, try to lift your arms as high up as you can, keeping them there for a count of ten seconds. Then bring them down and relax for ten seconds. Progress this exercise with one-pound hand weights in each hand, increasing the weight by one pound each time to eventually reach the five-pound level.

*Your goal:* one set of ten reps, holding for ten seconds, resting for ten seconds between each rep.

*What to watch out for:* If you find it too hard to lift your arms, try moving your arms farther from your head until you can lift your arms and hold the position. The closer your arms are to your head, the more difficult the exercise is. Only when your arms are almost touching your head should you then start using or increasing weight.

You can also do this exercise with one arm if you like, but I prefer that you start with two arms to balance out both of your sides.

## HOW DOES YOUR HIP MOVE?

Your hip is very important when it comes to running, and any changes to the way the hip moves can definitely cause knee pain. Tight hip muscles can alter the way you run and cause biomechanical changes to not only the position of the hip, but also to your pelvis, ankle, and knee. Most runners develop tight hip flexor and quad muscles if they haven't focused specifically on those areas before. A runner with tight hip flexors compensates: instead of keeping their legs staying in a straight, neutral alignment with both feet pointing forward, they rotate the foot outward, swinging the leg forward, and come back in quickly, like a forehand in tennis. This is because hip flexor and quad muscles have become short and tight, which prevents the full extension hip movement that your body needs in order to harness the power of your hip. I have seen many runners who don't bring their leg back in the motion, the leg always staying forward.

Other than losing that powerful hip extension movement—from which most of your power is generated—your front thigh muscles tighten up, generating less power as a result. This huge imbalance decreases your hip extension, preventing your leg from internally rotating to the middle. This opened-up position opens your hips too much, making you look as if you are dragging a dead tree branch every time you take a step. This consequently also makes your knee drop inward, causing the dreaded iliotibial (IT) band syndrome, as well as to osteoarthritis to the knee joint area. If you get this type of arthritis in your knee, it may stop your running cold.

You can buy the most expensive shoes out there with super-cushioned, motion-controlled support, but it won't help you. Restoring your strength in your hip extension by strengthening your glutes helps the biomechanics in your running. Some of the exercises that were mentioned in the previous chapter for working your glutes, including bridging, side-leg lifting, and stretching your quads and hip flexor muscles, definitely help. Also, try to sit as little as possible. I know that might sound like a joke but think about it: we all sit for long periods of time, whether doing our homework, surfing the Web, or working at our desks at work. We have become a society of sitting. We sit so much that our muscles, especially our glute muscles, have atrophied and become flat. It's as if those areas do not remember how to contract. They have memory loss. Bending forward is also why our hips tighten up. You know that stiff feeling when you stand up from a sitting position that makes you feel as if you might fall? Now you know where that comes from. We really need to start working those areas; if not, your running techniques, times, and efficiency will suffer.

## YOUR ANKLES

How many times have you rolled inward on your ankles and hoped the pain would go away if you just kept running? It's hard enough to run on the street on hard pavement, but how would it feel on an uneven surface, like sand or grass? I would guess that the initial pain and discomfort would only get worse.

If runners who get "rolled ankles" don't understand what's going on and how to transform their ankles from their weak link to a strong foundation, they risk jeopardizing their running season.

"Rolling your ankle" is another term for ankle sprain, usually involving the three outer ligaments of the ankle: the anterior talofibular ligament (ATF), calcaneofibular ligaments (CF), and the posterior talofibular ligament (PTF). One thing to know is that a ligament starts from a bone and finishes at a bone, so it cannot contract by itself. The most common ligament sprain is the ATF sprain, in which the ligament has been stretched, causing swelling and pain. It prevents you from walking properly. The structure that contracts is your tendons, because they start from your bones but connect into your muscles. One of the major muscles of the ankle involved in ankle sprains is the peroneal muscle, which runs along the outside of your shin. When your leg starts to roll in, these muscles are supposed to contract to stop the ankle from turning in. They are also involved in pushing your foot off the ground, along with your calf muscles. This is called plantarflexion. When your peroneal muscles become weak, it's only a matter of time before your ankle ligaments weaken, too.

The best way to start to strengthen these muscles is with calf raises, which strengthen the peroneal muscles, as well as the deep muscles of the leg, giving you a much better sense of strength and stability. Practicing one-leg balance exercises for about thirty seconds each time, starting with eyes open and then moving on to eyes closed, gives you the power that you need. There is no need to go to unstable surfaces like a bosu ball if you can't master one-foot balancing on a stable surface. You should always consult with a physical therapist, doctor, or health consultant to suggest an appropriate program to follow.

Another area often injured is the Achilles tendon. The tendon acts like spring-like cord, which is vital in walking, let alone running. Sometimes referred to as your heel cord, the Achilles tendon is a six-inch band of super-tough tendon that's strong enough to support your weight, help you jump and land, run at your top speed, and do so many other things that we take for granted. You'd think that we'd take care of something so important to us, keeping our Achilles tendon flexible and strong. Unfortunately, some of us don't like stretching our calf muscles, to which the tendon is attached. We love running on our thick-soled shoes for miles upon miles, not realizing that the tendon could stiffen up and tighten. And if we have weak knees that tend to drop inward while we run, that force pulls the Achilles tendons out of alignment, stressing and straining them. The tendons can take only so much before pain sets in. Then you start to compensate and alter your running pattern, or you stop running altogether. A proper stretching program makes the calves flexible, thereby enabling the proper foot and ankle mechanics, which allows your ankle to move properly and absorb and evenly disperse the forces going through your foot.

## COMPRESSION SLEEVE

There's a lot of controversy about whether compression sleeves are beneficial for runners. They're definitely helpful for blood circulation problems, especially those with varicose veins. One of the big uses for them is when runners have to take an airplane to a race. Has your foot ever throbbed after a race and a plane ride? A compression sock helps to control changes in pressure in your body, especially in your feet, due to changes in altitude. The great thing about compression socks is that they are inexpensive and can ease the pain and soreness that you might feel from aching joints or any sports-related soreness.

Compression sleeves have been shown to work the best when they are combined with treatments suggested by your physical therapist or other allied professional. The combination of the two helps to decrease some of the inflammation and irritation that you might experience. Many of you will find that your knees are better able to tolerate certain activities like walking, running, tennis, and golfing when wearing a compression sleeve or supportive brace. The compression sleeves not only alleviate some of the pain and discomfort, but they also provide you with an improved sense of knee stability. Try wearing a pair of compression socks after your run for a short time every day so that you can get used to them. Definitely wear them when you get on a plane. They could also be worn after high-intensity workouts that involve running. If you get calf cramps after long runs, compression socks help you to recover faster from training sessions.

## RUNNING TIPS

Here are some small but useful tips about how to prevent injury while running. One of the big reasons that runners get injured is the stride they take. Some runners tend to take bigger steps than necessary, or overstride.

When your foot continually lands in front of your center mass, you are overstriding. Your normal or ideal stride is the distance from where your foot hits the ground back to a straight invisible line down from your center of mass through the middle of your lower back.

Overstriding has been demonstrated to place additional, unnecessary pressure on your knees and body. You might have enough strength to absorb this additional stress, but it can cause pain in your joints. The other problem is that the longer the stride, the higher you jump in the air, and, therefore, the harder you land on the ground. This again creates more impact for your joints to absorb.

When you overstride, you straighten your knee, causing your heel to absorb all the impact and shock instead of your muscles. The shock is then transferred to the knee menisci, knee joint, and on to the hip and back joints. To know what your running cadence should ultimately be, count the number of right foot strikes in thirty seconds and multiply by four. Your number of right foot strikes should be between 145 and 190. An ideal range for most runners is between 170 and 190 strikes. As mentioned earlier, try to slowly reduce the amount of heel cushion in your shoe. This is called "drop" or "heel-toe offset" in shoe terms. If you're in twelve-millimeter drop shoes now—which is what most shoes are—try going with an eight millimeter drop when you buy your next pair of new shoes, eventually working your way to a six millimeter drop. A less cushioned heel discourages a huge, overstriding heel-strike pattern of landing. You'll notice that your new shoes have less structure and aren't as stiff, which means that your foot gets to work more naturally. You won't be depending so much on padding but on strengthening your foot muscles so that they can perform their natural movement.

Another thing that we should pay attention to is to practice running on different types of surfaces. I'm not suggesting running on only dirt or grass, but your foot and body should learn how to run on all sorts of surfaces, from the pavement on the road to sand and everything in between. Alternating between harder and softer terrain keeps you running and your legs fresh.

Research study after study has clearly shown that faster runners tend to run more miles. But how do you reach a higher mileage total without getting injured? The best way to do that is to add no more than 10 percent more miles from one week to the next. Remember that if you progress slowly but surely and control your road-running enthusiasm, you will reach your goals injury free.

Your baseline number should be the number of kilometers that you feel comfortable running every week. You shouldn't be out of breath when running at this pace. Please keep in mind that everybody's pace is different. A good starting point is to look at the distance you've been running during the last four to six months, then start increasing it by 10 percent per week. It should still be safe and comfortable at this level. Eventually, you can even increase it to 15 percent per week, but don't overdo it. If you pass your baseline by too much margin, bring it down. Try not to be a hero. You're trying to prevent injuries while still running more over time.

Here is something else you probably won't like, but it's a necessary evil: take a recovery week every four to six weeks. For example, if you're running forty kilometers per week with a five kilometer speed run and a ten-kilometer long run, a recovery week might be only a twenty to twenty-five kilometer run, a three kilometer speed run (or any other shorter run), and an eight kilometer longer run. Whatever you decide to do during your recovery week, it should be about 25 percent less than what you were running the previous week so that your body has a chance to catch up to your hard-running workouts.

## TREADMILL RUNNING VERSUS RUNNING OUTSIDE

The treadmills at our gym are always full. They may be the most popular piece of cardio equipment in any gym. So what's the difference between running indoors on the treadmill and enjoying a run outside? Although many experts say that outdoor running generally provides a better workout, the treadmill provides some benefits that you can't get by running outside.

Running on a treadmill can have some advantages. Here are some of the benefits:

- Less pounding on your joints: the shock-absorbing surface of the treadmill makes it easier on the knees, hips, and ankles than pounding the pavement. Less pounding allows you to run longer with less discomfort.
- You can stop whenever you want: if you run on a treadmill, you can stop any time you feel like it. You won't need to take the bus because you are so far from home. If you run outside and need to stop running (if you are getting muscle cramps, getting winded or just plain

tired), you may find yourself walking for a long time. If you're running inside on a treadmill and have completed your mileage, you can simply press the stop button. No long walks.

- You run faster: when working out on the treadmill, you tend to run at a faster pace than when running outside. This is due to the fact that the belt on the treadmill is moving and doing some of the work for you: you have the opportunity to increase your running speed. Treadmill running is a great way to learn how to increase your overall running speed.
- You have more control over your workout: it is easier to accomplish your workout goals using a treadmill than by running outside. You can still achieve your goal outside, but it is easier to press a button if you want to do interval training, run hills, or let the computer mix it up for you.
- You can multitask: running on the treadmill lets you catch up on the news of the day or watch your favorite sport or TV show, distracting you from the running. You can also multitask and still fit in your workout.
- You don't need to carry water: if you get thirsty while running outside, it might be difficult to find a water fountain or a local store to buy water. You can run with a water bottle, but it can be cumbersome and annoying. However, when you're running on a treadmill, your water bottle is right next to you, and you can take a sip whenever you want.
- You can easily track your stats: one of the great things about treadmill running is that the program tracks your distance and pace. You can monitor your heart rate, elevations, and other stats. Nowadays, we can also check our Apple watches, Garmin, or Fitbits, but if you don't have these, a treadmill provides all of these stats.

Here are some benefits of running outside:

- Running outside provides a better workout: you burn more calories running outside because it works your muscles much more. You have to move your legs rather than allowing the treadmill's belt to do it for you.
- You can start running at any time: you don't need to drive to your local gym to start running. Just put on your favorite running shoes and attire and enjoy the great outdoors!

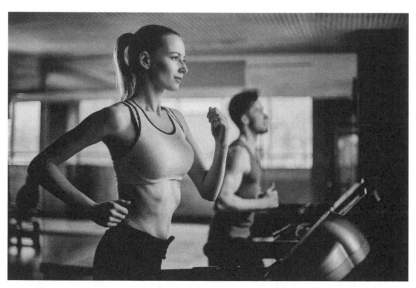

Woman Running on Treadmill. *Pressmaster, image from Bigstockphoto.com*

- Running outside is more interesting: running on a treadmill can be boring. Outside, you get to enjoy fresh air and beautiful scenery. When running at a steady pace, you often reach your destination without realizing that you ran that distance. Running outside distracts you from the mileage and leaves you in your own thoughts and peace of mind.
- Running outside offers more unpredictable surfaces than running on a treadmill: this provides the extra benefit of improving your balance and coordination. On uneven terrain, like grass or dirt, you have to work harder to counterbalance that crack in the pavement or mound in a field. Sand is a testing surface on which to run on, because it is difficult to push yourself forward. The softer the sand, the harder the run. Sand offers a challenging workout, testing your endurance and burning lots of calories.
- You feel accomplished: realizing that you ran a distance—whether five kilometers, ten kilometers, or from point A to point B—all by yourself on your own steam, provides a huge sense of achievement.
- Running outside is a great way to unplug (and reboot): there are very few ways left of getting away from all the noise of everyday life. Mobile phones and laptops mean that we are connected to everyone, all

of the time. Sometimes, it just feels good to get away from your boss, your coworkers, and even your family! Just a little bit of time all to yourself provides much-needed downtime.

## SAMPLE BODY TRAINING PROGRAM GEARED FOR RUNNING

Some runners reading this might say, "Why am I doing strength training when I'd rather concentrate on running?" Getting your body stronger and balanced prevents those nasty injuries that stop your progression. Runners, however, need a different type of strength-training program than your everyday iron-pumping individual. Instead of lifting heavy weights like bench presses and bicep curls in the attempt of lifting someone over their heads, runners should focus on targeting the key muscles that will keep them balanced.

If you want to perform at your full potential, you need to take a holistic approach to your running. This includes working on specific areas that you normally may not think of working on, like flexibility, balance, mobility, and strength. Studies have shown that strength training can improve your body structure by helping you to maintain or increase your lean body mass and decrease your percentage of body fat, helping you to look leaner and burn additional calories.

What follows is a sample training program that you can do to help you get stronger, expend less energy, and become much more efficient in your running. It might even help lower your time! Please keep in mind that this is an example of an exercise program. Also, this global program can be done if you do *not* have an existing knee injury. Please make sure that your doctor, physical therapist, or allied professional is advising you on the exercise program that's best for you.

**Sample Exercises**

*Week 1*

Clamshells 3 × 10
Side walk with tubing 3 × 10
Straight front leg lifts 3 × 10
Straight leg alphabet ×1
Bridging with two legs 3 × 10
Bridging with one leg 3 × 10
Side plank isometric hold 3 × 10 with 5-second hold

*Week 2*

>   Glutes medius up-down 3 × 10
>   Glutes medius circles 3 × 10
>   Straight side leg lifts 3 × 10
>   SLR (straight leg raise) side alphabet ×1
>   Step-ups 2 × 10
>   Step-downs 2 × 10
>   Wall squats 2 × 10 with 5-second hold
>   Side planks up-down 3 × 10
>   Balance on one leg, eyes open 3 × 10 with 30-second hold
>   Balance on one leg, eyes closed 3 × 10 with 30-second hold

Try alternating these routines weekly and incorporate them into your running schedule. After a month or so of this type of training, take a two-week break to allow your muscles to recuperate and grow. If you are sore from the training, please be sure to take a day or two off until you aren't sore and feel strong enough to continue.

What's most important with all of these exercises is feeling the contraction of the muscle that you are working on. If you are not feeling the muscle or muscles that you are trying to work on, then stop, reposition yourself, and try again. Sometimes, closing your eyes helps you to focus on feeling the muscle you are working. Make sure that the weight that you are working with is neither too heavy nor too light. Check your form and technique. You can try doing the exercise in front of a mirror or in front of someone else so that you are performing the exercise in the most precise way possible. If you find that your technique or your form is wrong, don't ignore it, because you would be simply cheating the movement and failing to gain the benefits you seek.

## SUMMARY

- The most common type of running injury is "runner's knee," or patellofemoral pain syndrome (PFPS).
- Foam rolling is a self-myofascial release (SMR) technique used by athletes and physical therapists to aid in muscle recovery.
- Foam rolling the IT band has not been shown to create significant, positive difference. The IT band is tough, fibrous, dense tissue; it is very hard to "loosen up." It is more beneficial to strengthen the

muscles that are attached to the IT band, which prevents spasming, and keep the area strong, flexible, and balanced.

- The two major muscles that are usually weak in runners and that could benefit greatly from a complete strengthening program are the gluteus medius and the vastus medialis muscles.
- There is no research that demonstrates that stability control and neutral position shoes are necessary for improving running performance. Strengthening the intrinsic muscles of your foot and your tibialis posterior muscle is a better route to follow. Also, keeping your gastrocnemius and soleus muscles flexible keeps your Achilles tendon loose and flexible, which allows better running flow.
- Take a recovery week every four to six weeks of running. Recuperation from intense runs only makes you stronger, because it allows your muscles to grow, it helps you to develop a stronger, more efficient nervous system, and it makes the organs and systems in your body work much more efficiently. You will also become less tired and full of energy to tackle the next phase.
- Overstriding puts a lot of pressure on your heels and increases impact and stress in your joints. Taking smaller, quicker steps transfers your weight more in line with your body's center of gravity and makes your running much more efficient.
- Running on different surfaces outside increases the strength in your limbs. Instead of running on hard pavement, alternate your running among pavement, grass, dirt, and even sand, which works your muscles in different ways, readying you for different obstacles that might come your way.
- Running on a treadmill burns fewer calories than running outside because the belt moves beneath you, but it is more convenient for some people because they can just press the stop button when their workout is finished. Running outside makes your muscles stronger, is less boring, and offers fresh air that you wouldn't get if you were stuck inside.

# 6

# Getting Your
# Knee into Super Shape!

Sometimes, you've got to make your work and workouts coexist.

—Jillian Michaels

Getting your knee stronger and more flexible by doing the rehabilitation exercises is one thing. But what can you do to continue this forward momentum when you go to the gym to work out or to participate in a class workout? How do you do a proper squat or deadlift? What kind of exercises and routines can you do to prevent future injuries from haunting you later? Remember that useful saying, one of many, by America's great revolutionary hero and statesman, Benjamin Franklin: "An ounce of prevention is worth a pound of cure." Strengthening your muscles around the knee joint area will protect you from getting injured by decreasing stressful forces that are placed on your knee. Now that you've done the hard and maybe lengthy work toward a cure, it's time to think about prevention: strength-building exercises to improve your stability and give you the confidence to do things you once thought you might never have the power to do again. I want you to make your legs—injured and noninjured—strong, fit, and active again. You want to return to your sport or favorite pastime without fearing about the pain returning.

## HOW DO YOU MAKE MUSCLES STRONGER?

The fact of the matter is that the body, which is an amazingly ingenious creation, can adapt extremely well to forces and stresses placed upon it.

Maybe you've noticed people working out in the gym for months and months, applying themselves assiduously, yet never achieving any noticeable bodily changes. They look the same after their fiftieth workout as they looked after their first. Why? Those people almost certainly do the same routine—comprised of the exact same exercises and lifting the same amount of weight during every workout they do—workout after workout, week after week, month after month. It stands to reason that if you keep doing the same thing, you'll get the same result. If you change nothing, you will never see any change in your body nor in your level of strength. Why would you?

The secret to making your muscles stronger is understanding the body's efficiency. It does what is demanded of it but nothing more; that's how it conserves the energy it needs to power you through your day—and through your life. So if you do one set of hamstring curls with fifteen-pound weights for months on end, your body "understands" that it needs only to be strong enough to lift fifteen pounds—not an ounce more. That's its point of stability, and it will stay at that strength level until a greater force or stiffer demand is made upon it. There's even a name for this expression of bodily efficiency and stability: general adaptation syndrome. Simply put, the body has adapted to the exercise demands placed on it to the point that, as far as your muscles are concerned, no change is needed.

So what do you do to gain strength in your body? It's simple: you give your muscles a reason to raise their level of efficiency and stability. I like to think of it as a process of shock and awe: you change some element in your exercise routine, introducing a behavior or practice your body is not used to that, as a result, surprises the muscles and jolts them into responsive action. You were using fifteen pounds on the hamstring machine? What happens when you raise the weight to twenty pounds? You were accustomed to doing three sets of eight reps? Try three sets of ten reps or maybe five sets of eight. You used to rest for one minute between sets? Try limiting your rest to thirty seconds and see what happens.

For one thing, you'll feel the difference in each case, even if you made only a small adjustment. Accustomed to the fifteen pounds, your body struggles to lift twenty pounds. Your muscles simply aren't ready for that change. Remember that they had adapted to fifteen pounds, so they are shocked at this new demand being made on them and awed that it's a full five pounds heavier. Your muscles need to readapt, and that's exactly what they do. During the rest time you give your body, the cells of the muscles, the tissue and fibers, and the energy centers of the muscles expand to meet the demand placed on them by the new weight. Keep it up and over time the muscles adapt upward to the new standard you have set.

The same thing happens if you increase the number of sets or reduce the length of your rest breaks, even if you're still lifting fifteen pounds. Increasing the number of sets requires more endurance; taking shorter rest breaks makes it tougher for the body to recover. Both actions make it harder to lift the same weight again, and the new demands stimulate your muscles to get stronger for the next time.

Of course, the reverse is also true. "Use it or lose it" isn't just a cute quote; it's a scientific reality where muscles are concerned. You can work your way up to a routine of five sets of twenty-pound curls with ten reps per set, and as soon as you switch to fifteen-pound weights, or only three sets, or eight reps per set, you shock your muscles to adapt downward, and they shrink to the lesser demands placed on them.

So as you read this chapter and fashion a program to get your knees strong and flexible and to keep them that way for life, it's important to remain mindful of these realities. It's also essential to start slowly, easing back into your exercise program, and keep at it.

## YOUR SUPER-KNEE WORKOUTS

This chapter contains three workouts I've devised specifically for people returning to the gym after a knee injury or for those want to get stronger and more balanced in order to work on their favorite sport. Two of the workouts are at beginner level; both are for easing back into flat-out, intensive muscle work. Why two beginner workouts? It's a hedge against boredom, and boredom is a hedge against neglecting your workouts. I want those who are returning to gym work to stay at this beginner level for at least six months; in preparing two different workouts for those six months, I'm giving you the ability to switch from one to the other. If people grow bored with their exercises, they tend to take shortcuts. They try to speed things up, and all too often, they move on to a more advanced level, even if they are not fully ready to do so. In this case, if you get bored with one set of beginner exercises, there's another, and that means there's no excuse for playing fast and loose with the six-month ease-in period. But once you've spent half a year doing the beginning workouts, workout number three takes it up a notch.

Beginner or advanced, easing in or steady state, the purpose of these exercise workouts is to grow stronger—specifically, to better balance your muscle strength and flexibility in your knees, hips, ankles, and feet. All of these joints working together do all the lifting, jumping, and running. You will be able to perform at your best any way you decide you need to do it, whether up, down, or even sideways. Each of these three workouts provides a collection of exercises you can choose from to build and maintain strong, powerful knees. Repeat each exercise a number of times, which are counted as repetitions of the movement.

The first question everyone wants to know is how often to do the exercises and how much weight to use. Both are good questions, so let's turn to the answers now.

## HOW OFTEN SHOULD I WORK OUT?

Based both on research I have seen and my own experience as a physical therapist working with a varied population, I recommend that you do your super-knee workout routine no more than two times a week, leaving at least a couple of rest days between workouts. In other words, you can work out every third day or so. The reason this differs from an upper body workout like my shoulder workout is that you need your legs to get around walking, climbing up and down stairs, and so on. Even though that might not sound like a lot of effort, your legs are still working on strength and balance during their everyday activities. Muscles normally get stronger after a good night's sleep, hopefully seven or eight hours. When you are training, you are actually microtearing the muscle. New muscle, cartilage, and other fibers are laid down, and this begins to make your muscles bigger and stronger. You are also giving your muscles, the surrounding tissues, and nerves the rest they need.

Okay, sometimes you miss a workout. You thought you had time to hit the gym this evening, but then your boss asks you to stay late, a friend calls with a free ticket to that concert you've been dying to go to, or you feel a cold coming on and figure you should get home to bed. Whatever the reason, it's a reminder that we don't live in a perfect world where nothing ever interferes with our plans.

Sometimes, you miss the next workout, as well: the cold lingers, the boss again asks you to stay late, or there's a movie you're just dying to see. Now you've missed two workouts in a row, and the tendency is to feel that you've blown it, it's all too much, and you might as well quit try-ing to maintain a regular schedule of workouts. But that kind of thinking is always a mistake, so please don't quit. Even two workouts a week will give you great results, almost as good as training three times a week. This is a case where consistency is more important than perfectly adhering to a schedule. Try for the former, and don't worry if you don't achieve the latter. The results you need and want come from keeping at it, not from being perfect, which no one is.

On the other side of the coin, let me remind you again of the lesson learned earlier in this book: working out more often and more intensely will *not* make you stronger faster. Unfortunately, the body does not work that way. If you trained every day, your body never gets a chance to rest and grow; without such rest, you simply become more vulnerable to in-jury, and you further postpone the day when you get better and stronger.

## HOW MUCH WEIGHT SHOULD I START WITH?

Clearly, there is no single straightforward answer to this question. We are all different. Some people are naturally stronger in some areas and weaker in others, so it's a matter of trial and error for each of us. But here's the key: aim to feel the muscle working, not straining. Too much weight can compromise proper form and technique; too little weight won't consti-tute a workout.

So how do you measure what's too much and what's too little? My general rule of thumb is that the "correct" weight is one in which you can comfortably do eight repetitions but start to strain at more than ten repetitions. At the very least, when your last rep feels difficult to do, that's probably your limit or one rep over your limit.

Now that you have gotten the exercises from our previous chapters, I wanted to supplement your strength-building program with some great exercises that you can incorporate at the gym. These exercises definitely help to improve the strength and stability needed to give you the confi-dence to do things that you didn't think you would ever have the power to do again!

All of the exercises here are weight-training exercises using dumbbells, barbells, or cables. In general, dumbbells provide greater range of motion than a barbell, and they also make you work harder, because dumbbells stay straight only because you stabilize them. Another plus, of course, is that it's a bit faster and easier to let a dumbbell drop than a barbell, should it become necessary to do so. The barbell, on the other hand, offers the advantage of a fixed and stable weight; there's no deviation, and that makes the barbell easy to work with. Cable machines offer flexibility and complexity—the arms can go in different directions at once in a controlled and stable manner, for example—that make it extremely utilitarian. They also provide a unique "feel" in the kind of resistance you're up against.

So it's useful and indeed desirable to use all three of these technologies in your workouts if you can. It's particularly useful to switch from one to another. Variety is as good for the body as for the mind. Mixing it up not only keeps you from getting bored with your exercise routine, but it's also a great way to challenge your muscles. That's the objective of these routines. Some of the exercises in the routines may be new to you, and that's a good thing. Remember: shock and awe are good for your muscles. Accustomed to training a certain way with a certain weight, they need a jolt to get stronger and tougher. Once you have figured out which exercises you find easy and which are hard, start your workout with the hard ones first. Your energy level is at its highest at the beginning of a workout; by the end of a workout session, your energy is draining, your mind starts to wander, and you're in danger of losing focus. So it's best to do the tougher exercises first, when they will seem easier to you. With the easier work at the end, you'll find out that you can keep going longer, as well.

## WILL I NEED TO DO THESE EXERCISES FOREVER IN ORDER TO PREVENT FUTURE INJURY?

This is a question I am frequently asked, and although no one can predict with certainty what may happen to an individual in the future, research clearly shows that quad and hamstring muscles that start strong require less "repair" after an injury than muscles that have not been exercised. Once you meet your strength goal for your quads, you need only train once a week to maintain the gain in strength. There is a catch, however: you have to exercise at the same intensity consistently, every time you are working out the knee area, so keep that in mind as you perform these exercises and work your way back to full strength.

The lesson is clear: exercise is the best way to achieve and maintain rock-solid knees for life.

One final but important note: if you are not sure whether a particular exercise is right for you, be sure to ask your doctor or health professional. Only when you are confident that an exercise can help you will you be motivated to do it, to do it correctly, and thereby to become stronger. You will feel a whole lot better and your knee will thank you!

Let's move on to the exercises.

## SQUATS

When most people hear the word *squat*, they probably think of a big guy at the gym holding a barbell on his back, lifting some heavy weight. I think we sometimes forget that we squat during the day, whether sitting in the bathroom or picking something off the floor. The squat exercise is one of the hall-of-fame exercises along with the deadlift and bench press that builds strength, power, and mobility. Practicing squats can help build your weak legs and glute muscles and start reversing and strengthening your hunched back and weak abs resulting from all the sitting that you do daily. The main muscles used in squats are quads, hamstrings, and glute muscles, but to some degree, you are working all the muscles from your abs to your feet.

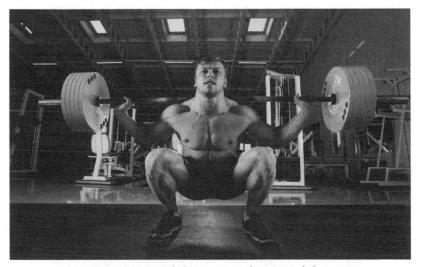

Man Doing Squats. *Takoburito, image from Bigstockphoto.com*

So how far down should you squat? Until your thighs are parallel to the floor, so that you don't get hurt, right? Well, I believe that you should squat fully, not just to the parallel level. If you do not have a preexisting problem, like osteoarthritis or an injury, it is actually beneficial for an everyday individual working on an unloaded deep squat, which is defined as "resting posture of maximal hip and knee flexion where the posterior thighs are in contact with the calves and the heels remain flat on the floor."[1]

Some other research studies demonstrate that performing a full-range or deep squat does *not* increase the risk of developing osteoarthritis (OA) of the knee.[2] However, other studies have shown that prolonged squatting, which was classified for about thirty minutes a day, followed by deep squatting causes knee osteoarthritis.[3] The practical and obvious question is, how many of us do deep squatting for thirty minutes a day? My guess is very few of us. We North Americans generally spend most of our day sitting in front of our computers with our hips and knees flexed at 90 degrees; we stand, walk, maybe run, and then go to bed after a long day. I don't think most of us practice bending past 90 degrees of flexion, though I believe we should. This is our full range of motion, and we should have full strength in our full range of motion. It's like performing a bench press or push-up only half of the way or doing a bicep curl part of the way for fear of getting injured. My four-year-old daughter stays in a deep squat to pick flowers from the garden. If it's good enough for her, when she doesn't know any better, it should be good for all of us.

Also, our lower extremity joints have special fluids in them called synovial fluid and hyaluronic acid. These fluids are needed for proper joint and cartilage health. These fluids help the joints reduce friction between different bone surfaces, provide shock absorption, and carry much-needed nutrients to the layer of cartilage on the surface of each of your joints. It has been shown that all synovial joints need movement as well as compression to keep cartilage healthy.[4]

One of the reasons that people cannot perform a deep squat properly is that they lack ankle and hip flexibility. Working on increasing ankle flexibility by doing standard calf stretches against a wall helps. Focus on increasing your hip flexion range of motion by working on the flexibility of your quads, hip flexors, and all the muscles around your hips. Mechanically you are at your weakest at the bottom range of the squat because you have to maintain control moving downward and then stop and change directions, all with proper form. It is not easy at all, but with patience, you can develop incredible power and strength. At deep squat levels, you start to develop your gluteus maximus, as well as the difficult-to-recruit VMO muscle of the quads, which gets stimulated as you come out of the squat.

For older people who can't squat deeply, doing a chair squat—that is, squatting down until the bottom touches the chair and then coming up—can produce strength in the hip and knee extensors, as well as the plantar flexors of the foot. Doing squats with your body weight alone is an excellent place to start. You don't need a heavy bar, just good mechanics.

## Do's and Don'ts of a Squat

To perform a squat with your own body weight, put your arms straight out in front of you, parallel to the ground. Keep your spine in a simple, neutral position. Try not to round your back but also don't hyperextend and over accentuate the natural arch of your back. Keep your chest out.

Look at your feet. The weight of your feet should be felt on the heels and the balls of your feet, as if you were stuck to the ground. You should be able to move your toes freely throughout the entire movement. If you find that your toes are trying to grip the floor instead of staying loose, you might need to work on building strength in your feet.

Take a deep breath, keep your body strong and tight, bend forward at your hips, and stick your butt out. Send your hips backward as you begin to bend your knees. Practice sticking your hips back first, rather than just bending your knees. Look straight ahead at a spot on the wall, not down at your feet. Your back is nice and straight with your neutral spine, and your chest and shoulders are up. Keep looking straight ahead at that spot on the wall.

When you start squatting downward, do not allow your knees to pass your feet—specifically, your big toe. New squatting recruits let their knees fall inward, causing poor biomechanics and lots of stress and discomfort of the knee joints. Focus on pushing your feet into the ground and keeping the knees out so that they fall in line with the feet. When they start to come inward, push them out to be in line with, but not wider than, your feet. Think about it like this: if you drew a straight line down from the middle of your kneecaps to your feet, the line should end between your second and fourth toes. Make sure that your knees are in the proper position.

Squat down until your hip joint is lower than your knees or as low as you can go. Depending on the size of your thighs, your squat may appear more shallow than it actually is. You can go deeper than this; however, if your thighs are less than parallel, it's a partial squat. Once you have reached your rock bottom, it's time to come back straight up. Keeping proper form, breathe out through your mouth and push hard through your heels. Try to keep your knees the same way you did on the way down, and squeeze your butt at the top of the movement to ensure you're using your glutes. Speed is also important. Try to come down slowly, for about three seconds, and come up quickly, which should take about one second. When you are at the deepest part of the squat, try not to bounce up, but come to a complete stop before starting to stand up. That way you are not using momentum, but you have proper control.

## Common Mistakes

### Letting the Knees Fall In

I believe the number-one problem with squats is when the knees fall inward. This is probably due to weak glutes, namely your gluteus medius, as well as an imbalance of strength between your inner and outer thighs. Most of the time, your outer thighs are stronger than your inner thighs. Weak calves and no strength in your feet also contribute. When your knees fall into each other during a squat, it puts a lot of stress and pressure on your knee ligaments, especially your anterior cruciate ligament (ACL). This helps to explain the proliferation of surgeries on the knee ligaments. However, correcting these mistakes isn't as simple as mentally forcing your knees into the proper position. You need to strengthen all the muscles we've discussed to create a better balance of strength among all your muscles, front and back, left and right.

### Lowering to 90 Degrees or Less

As stated before, if you don't squat to your full range of motion—meaning all the way down, not partway—you won't fully contract your glutes or the upper hamstrings muscles. If you aren't sure that you can perform the entire move, start by practicing some squats in front of a knee-high box or step. Lower your body until your behind just barely touches the box and then push back up. Once that is comfortable, try a lower level.

*Too Little Arch in Your Lower Back*

Your lower back naturally has a slight S-shape to it. If you are sitting in a poor position all day, your back flattens and loses the S-curve in that area. This puts a lot of weight on an area that can't fully absorb it if you have a limited range of motion in your lower back. Try bending backward to help improve the range of motion in your lower back. To shore up your lower-back strength, try performing some traditional deadlifts. I also highly suggest that you contract your glute muscles before you start your squat. It helps improve your form. Your chest should be up and your shoulders should be back. Your body should stay in this position the entire time. You don't want your shoulders to round forward, but you also don't want to hyperextend your back, either. Keep your spine in a neutral position throughout the movement.

*Lifting Less Weight Than You Can Handle*

If you complete your squats with light dumbbells in hand, you might want to consider reaching for something heavier, especially women. There's a misconception among women that they should perform a lot of repetitions with minimal weight if they want to slim their legs. However, if you don't lift an adequate and challenging amount of weight, you aren't going to tone anything. Plus, when you lift heavier weights, you burn more calories. You don't need to lift a house, just enough weight to feel difficulty between reps eight through ten. You'll get stronger legs because of it.

*Improper Foot Positioning*

It's very important to keep your heels flat on the ground throughout your squat. You should be pushing the power through your heels, and to do that, your feet must be flat. Although some of your weight may be on the balls of your feet, you never want the balls of your feet or your toes to bear the entire weight. You should be able to lift your toes up off the ground and wiggle them at any point, and it shouldn't affect your squat.

**One-and-a-Quarter Squats**

This is an exercise that works your vastus medialis oblique (VMO) muscle, that hard-to-reach area that's part of the vastus medialis muscle.

Developing that area helps stabilize your knee and balances out the naturally strong vastus lateralis. The VMO quickly wastes away during an injury, perhaps because it does a lot of eccentric work as a shock absorber. The stronger your VMOs, the less time it takes you to switch from eccentric to concentric phases of both sprinting and jumping. The VMO is stimulated at the bottom of a squat, as you are coming out of it.

Squat down for a five-second count until you hit your bottom position, holding it for one second, then coming up a quarter of the way at a slow and deliberate pace, then going all the way back down, under control, until the hamstrings cover the calves. Then come up fully. That counts as one rep.

*Your goal*: one set of ten reps, eventually graduating to three sets of ten reps. Only when you are strong enough can your progress to using weights.

*What to watch out for*: This is a difficult exercise to perfect. Many people underestimate how hard it is without any weights. Try pushing through your heels as you come upward to get a better contraction through your legs.

### Front Squats

The front squat, cousin to the squat and sometimes called the back squat, is an exercise in which you place the barbell in front of you instead of on your back. This type of squat makes your quadriceps muscles work much harder than your hamstrings, and you need abdominal strength to keep your body in an upright position. Most people lift more weight doing front squats and may find that keeping the rack position of the bar difficult; front squats are not done as frequently as they should. Of course, this is a huge mistake for anyone looking to build power and strength, correct muscle imbalances, and, as an added benefit, get some good-looking abs.

Start by moving under the bar with your arms and grasp it with a closed overhand grip slightly wider than shoulder width. Put the bar evenly on top of your front deltoids and collarbone. Take your thumb and pinky finger out from under the bar and keep a relaxed, open palm with three fingers under the bar. Take a couple of steps backward. Inhale and hold that breath toward the bottom of the movement to maintain intra-abdominal tightness. Start bending your hips and knees slowly as you go

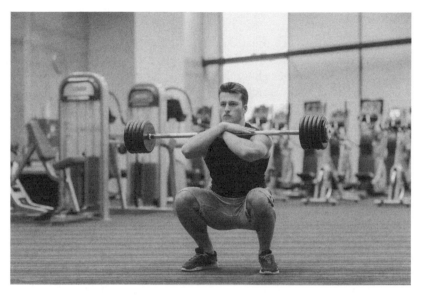

Front Squat. *Dolgachov, image from Bigstockphoto.com*

into the movement. Remember to push your knees outward as you squat down, paying attention to your proper alignment. Once you get to the bottom of the movement, be sure to squeeze the elbows up and inward. Focus on keeping your elbows up at the bottom of the lift.

Once your thighs are parallel with the ground, push yourself upward but keep your heels flat on the floor and your knees in a straight line with your feet. Halfway up, exhale and power through with the glutes and core braced until you reach the top position.

*Your goal*: three sets of ten reps, breaking for thirty seconds in between sets.

*What to watch out for*: Sometimes people may have great mobility and flexibility but don't focus on the right cues while they're doing front squats and mistakes happen. Common problems include dropping the elbows, the torso falling forward, not going deep enough in the squat, and allowing your knees to collapse inward or to flare out way too much. Mistakes cause a poor-quality squat with less-than-ideal weight coupled with knee or other joint pain, which makes you not want to do the exercise anymore.

## Hack Squats

The purpose of a hack squat is to develop the lower part of your thigh near your patella. The hack squat exercise primarily targets your quadriceps, but also works your glutes, hamstrings, calves, and lower back—it's a complete lower body exercise. The hack squat offers support and protection to your lower back that free-weight standing squats do not. It also allows you to take a much narrower stance when performing the movement without the complications of being unbalanced, since the machine provides stability. It's probably most advantageous to start strengthening your knees with the hack squat until you have the strength, balance, and stability needed to use the freestanding squat rack.

Using a full range of motion, bend your knees all the way down to the floor and push yourself back up until your legs are almost straight without locking them. Always keep your back and head against the padding, your shoulders under the shoulder pads, and hold on to the handles, which are usually near the shoulder pads or at your sides near the hips. Put your legs in a slightly forward angle from where your upper body is. This keeps the knees from sticking out past your feet, which takes pressure off your knees. From your starting position, push up to release the safety bar and move the safety handles to free the sliding mechanism. Keep your legs straight without locking the knees. Lower the bar slowly until your thighs and lower legs form an angle slightly less than 90 degrees. Check that your knees are above your feet and not past them. Then push through your heels to power yourself back to the starting position. Repeat for the desired number of repetitions.

*Your goal*: three sets of ten repetitions, breaking for thirty seconds between sets.

*What to watch out for*: Placing your feet properly is very important in executing the hack squat well. If you practice good form, the exercise is safe and won't harm your knees. Always point your toes slightly outward when planting your feet on the platform. Doing so allows your quadriceps muscles to engage more and takes pressure off the medial collateral ligament in the knees. Do not point your toes straight ahead or you risk overloading knee cartilage. The hack squat can be performed using various stance widths. If any particular stance causes discomfort when performing the exercise, adjust the width of your stance.

Although you might be tempted to use a lot of weight, do not do so if it affects your technique or causes injury. You'll produce great results if you slowly increase weight while always maintaining proper positioning.

Machine hack squats require strong vastus medialis muscles and extremely good knee stability to be truly effective.

You might find machine hack squats more effective when you progressively raise up on the balls of the feet while coming down. Once the bottom position is reached, concentrate on pushing off the ball of the feet to further stimulate the vastus medialis muscles. As you ascend, progressively lower your heels to the platform.

## DEADLIFTS

Deadlifts and squats are two of the most important lower body exercises. In my opinion, the deadlift is one of the most effective exercises for developing the posterior chain of your body, which is normally the weak link, even for athletes. Since it's a full-body exercise that recruits a lot of muscle mass, the deadlift also builds muscle in many places simultaneously. It's also one of the few exercises that works on the lower back muscles, the gluteus maximus, and the hamstrings, which are groups of muscles that are often neglected in the weight room.

### What's the Proper Way to Perform a Deadlift?

Try this approach: place both feet under the bar so that the middle of each foot is under the bar. Maintain a hip-width stance with your toes pointing slightly away from the middle at about 15 degrees turnout. Grab the bar with both of your hands about shoulder width apart. Arms are vertical from the front view, hanging just outside your legs. Now, start bending your knees down toward the floor until you find that your shins are touching the bar. At this point, lift your chest up and keep your back nice and straight, no hunching. Keep your hips forward, and without squeezing your shoulder blades, drop your hips. Holding the bar in your hands, try to stand up, pulling the bar with you. Make sure the bar is not swinging; keep it close to your legs.

You have completed a repetition when you have completely locked your hip and knees. Now you can bring the weight back to the floor by pushing your hips back and bending your legs when the bar reaches the knee area again, but not before that point. If you try to bend your knees first, you'll hit them with the bar, and that will hurt—trust me!

*Your goal*: three sets of ten repetitions.

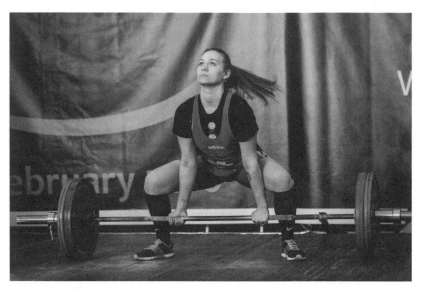

Girl Performing Deadlift. *sportpoin74, image from Bigstockphoto.com*

*What to watch out for:* Bouncing the barbell off the floor, which might cause an injury. Start every rep from a dead stop, with no momentum. Good cues that you can use to visualize the deadlift might be thinking of pressing the floor away from you, like you would do if you were performing a leg press. Think also about squeezing your gluteal muscles and driving your hips forward, not about lifting the bar upward. This helps you to keep the bar straight and to lock your knees more easily.

Hand grip is also important. There are two major types of grip when performing the deadlift: overhand and alternate. With the overhand grip, both palms of the hands face the floor with the thumbs underneath the bar. The problem with this type of grip is that your grip might weaken and slip when using heavier weights. I don't want you to drop the weight and hurt yourself. This is the main reason why I prefer the alternative grip, which is an overhand/underhand type of grip. With this method, one palm faces the ceiling, and the other faces the ground. This position decreases the chances of the bar slipping out of your hands. If you want to get a better grip, use wrist straps or go completely old school and use chalk like powerlifters used to do. Any method is OK with me.

Make sure your back stays straight in any deadlifting movement. Focus on keeping the chest out and your chin up, with eyes focused straight ahead, not looking down to the ground. Try not to jerk the bar up your thigh. The movement should be smooth from top to bottom. Do not allow your knees to bend inward during the lift. Same rule as with the squat: don't go crazy with the weights. Go slowly and methodically. Concentrate on proper technique and form with light weights; you'll be able to lift heavier weights more easily if you maintain proper form.

## HAMSTRING CURLS

Hamstring curls are one of the best ways of strengthening your hamstring muscles, which are located on the opposite side of your quadriceps on the back of your leg. Strong hamstrings prevent knee ligament tears, especially of the ACL. There are lots of ways of strengthening your hamstring muscles through different curl positions: lying down, sitting, or standing.

### Lying Hamstring Curls

Start by lying down on the lying leg curl machine with your face toward the machine. Fix your feet under the foot pad, resting the pad over your ankles. Make sure that the foot pad is just above your heels and not on your calves. If there are handles on the machine, you may hold them if you like. Keep your back flat, and do not arch your spine. Curl your legs upward by bending your knees so that your hamstrings are fully contracted. Try holding the position for one second before slowly letting your legs return to the starting position.

*Your goal*: three sets of ten repetitions, breaking for thirty seconds between sets.

*What to watch out for*: Try keeping your hips on the bed when curling the weight in order to feel the contraction properly. Also, as mentioned earlier, the resistance should be at the top of your heel, not at midcalf. A variation to work the hamstring curl is to superset the exercise, which is doing two exercises in one: hamstring curls with the toes pointed out in a plantar-flexed position and then with the toes pulled back in a dorsiflexed position. This is a unique way of getting some more reps out of the exercise. Hamstring curls with toes pointed is much harder to do, so you can reach fatigue on that variation much more quickly, but instead of stopping, with a simple flick of your feet to toes-pointing-toward-you position, your calves now flex and help as you continue to perform more reps. This way, you can really get a burn of the hamstring muscles.

### Seated Hamstring Curls

The seated hamstring curl is basically a hamstring curl but in a sitting position. I have been asked, why perform it when you can do the lying hamstring curl instead? The reason is that the lying hamstring curl focuses primarily on working the outer part of the hamstrings, or the bicep femoris muscle, whereas seated leg curls work the inner two thirds of the hamstrings, the semimembranosus and semitendinosus muscles. This is very important if you want the full benefit of strengthening the hamstring muscle.

Adjust the machine lever to fit your height and sit on the machine with your back against the back-support pad. Place the back of your lower leg on top of the padded lever (just a few inches under the calves) and secure the lap pad against your quads, which should be just above your knees. Then grasp the side handles on the machine as you point your toes straight (you can also use either of the other two stances mentioned earlier), ensuring that the legs are fully straight, right in front of you. This is the starting position.

As you breathe out, bring the machine lever as far as possible from your hamstrings by bending at your knees. Keep your torso stable without moving throughout the movement. Hold the contracted position for a second and slowly let the bar down to the starting position.

*Your goal*: three sets of ten repetitions, breaking for thirty seconds between sets.

*What to watch out for*: Try not to use so much weight that it causes you to swing and jerk your leg around, as this can injure your lower back and cause a hamstring strain or even a tear. You can always try a variation of the exercise; you'll feel different areas working depending on which way your foot is pointing.


### LUNGES

A lot of people are afraid of doing lunges. They've heard stories that they cause knee pain and discomfort. However, they are great for building mass and strength. You can do lunges anywhere you are, and you'll feel the burn and the benefit in no time at all in the form of shapely, strong legs and a well-defined glute region if you do them properly. I'll explain how to do them so that you don't put unwanted pressure and strain on your joints.

Start by making sure that your upper body stays straight, with your shoulders back and relaxed, not hunched over. Keep your chin up. Pick a point on the wall in front of you to stare at so that you don't keep looking down at your feet, because that's where the trouble starts. Always tighten your abs through the movements, keeping them strong.

Move forward with one leg, lowering your hips until both of your knees are at or around a 90-degree angle with the floor. Make sure your front knee is directly above your ankle, not pushed out too far forward, and ensure that the heel of your other knee is not touching the floor. Keep the weight in your heels as you push back up to the starting position.

*Your goal*: three sets of ten reps, breaking for thirty seconds between reps.

*What to watch out for*: Lunges have a reputation for causing discomfort in the knees, and most people avoid them altogether. Some of the reasons for this can be explained. One of the big reasons is muscle imbalances

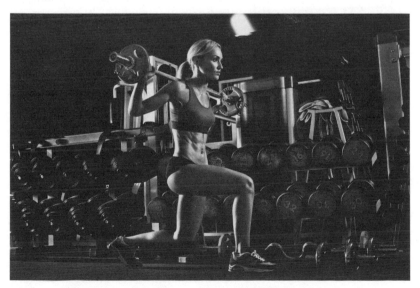

Lunges. *tankist, image from Bigstockphoto.com*

in the leg. Most people have their power in their legs located in their quadriceps muscle. The dominance of the quadriceps over the weaker hamstring and glutes muscles creates an imbalance of the lower body during lunging, because overusing the quadriceps causes a forward shift of the hips. This forward motion shifts the center of gravity forward and places more stress on the knees. When your muscles are more balanced in strength—quads with hamstrings, as well as glutes with calves—and you are aligned properly rather than leaning forward, you develop great power and strength.

Another reason for discomfort is lack of flexibility. If you have tight quadriceps and hip flexor muscles, they can pull on the tendons around your knee, causing some discomfort and pain when performing lunges. Tight muscles around your knee may also inhibit hip and knee movement and increase pressure in your knee joint, leading to discomfort. Warming up and stretching tight muscles before lunging can help reduce discomfort and make you feel the burn of your muscles!

## STEP UPS

Step ups are a great exercise to improve your strength and functionality, and they're not your standard way of doing an exercise. This exercise will definitely help you climb up and down stairs.

Take the bar (or dumbbells), put it on your shoulders in the high bar position, and step up on a bench with one leg. Bring the other leg all the way up to a 90-degree angle, then step back down to the floor with the same leg, switching legs the next time you step up.

For a tougher version of this exercise, try this: Start by stepping onto a bench with your right foot. Straighten your knee to stand on the bench while lifting your other leg so that your hip and knee are both at 90-degree angles. Keeping your right foot flat on the bench, bend your right knee as you lower your left foot to tap the floor with your left toes but without putting your weight onto your left foot. This completes one rep. Press through your right heel as you straighten your right knee to stand on the box. Not an easy exercise to do, but you'll feel those muscles working.

*Your goal:* three sets of ten repetitions, breaking for thirty seconds in between sets.

*What to watch out for:* Keeping your leg straight as you push your leg upward. Try pushing through your heels to get a better contraction. Make sure that your knee is aligned with your toe.

## LEG PRESSES

Leg presses on a machine are another great way to build mass and strength in your thighs. One of the great things about the leg press is that there's a lot less pressure on your lower back because you're seated and not standing, so you can use the weight that you want without worrying if your lower back can support it, as with a squat. Also with a leg press, you're pressing up instead of squatting down. The leg press machine allows more control of the amount of weight you can use than squats, which is great if you already have bad knees. Maintaining proper form on the leg press can only help you get stronger.

Sitting down on the leg press machine, position your feet on the platform directly in front of you at a medium stance. Remove the safety bars by lowering them down. Hold the weighted platform in place and press through your heels on the platform until your legs are fully extended in front of you, being careful not to fully lock your knees. Your abs and the legs should come to a 90-degree angle on the machine. This is your beginning point for the exercise. Then slowly lower the platform until your upper and lower legs make a 90-degree angle.

To reduce some of the stress on your knees, the leg press can done in an inclined position. Put the weights onto the foot platform and draw them down by bending your knees and pushing it back up. When you use the weight plates for resistance, it allows you to use as much or as little weight as you can tolerate. Using incline leg presses to strengthen your quadriceps provides the bonus of developing knee support. Try doing this type of exercise before you start your squats. The leg press is essentially a reverse squat, with the resistance load entirely on your legs rather than on your lower back. This is an exercise that offers the benefits of a squat but without stressing your lower back and knees.

*Your goal*: three sets of ten repetitions, breaking for thirty seconds between sets.

*What to watch out for*: To avoid injuring yourself when working on the incline leg press, make sure that your knees are always pointing forward and not flaring out and that your feet are flat on the footplate during the exercise. It's OK if your heels come off the footplate occasionally, but you should try to maintain full contact with the footplate as much as possible. When your legs are extended at the top of the move, make sure that your knees do not fully lock. As you lower the weight back down, do it slowly without allowing your quadriceps to touch your abdominal area.

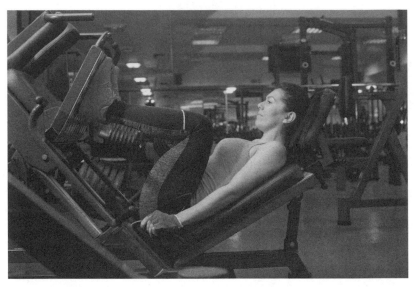

Woman Doing Leg Press Begin. *Creative Family, image from Bigstockphoto.com*

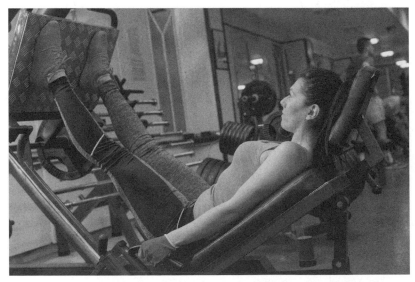

Woman Doing Leg Press End. *Creative Family, image from Bigstockphoto.com*

## WORKOUTS

Here are some sample workouts that can get your knees in tip-top shape!

### Routine 1

1. Squats 3 × 10
2. Lying hamstring curls 3 × 10
3. One-and-a-quarter squats: 2 × 10
4. Lunges 2 × 10
5. Quadriceps stretch 3 × 10 with 1-minute hold

### Routine 2

1. Deadlift 3 × 10
2. Leg presses 3 × 10
3. Step ups: 2 × 10
4. Seated hamstring curls 2 × 10
5. Hamstring stretch 3 × 10 with 30- to 60-second hold

### Routine 3

1. Hack squats 3 × 10
2. Calf raises 3 × 10
3. Front squats 2 × 10
4. Lying hamstring curls 2 × 10
5. Calf stretch 3 × 10 with 30-to 60-second hold

## GETTING YOUR KNEE READY FOR YOUR SPORT

We all have a favorite sport that we love to play. For some, it might be playing soccer, going for a lay-up in basketball, or spiking a volleyball. Whatever gives you that passion to play, having strong and balanced knees, hips, and ankles not only allows you to play your sport more efficiently, but it also greatly decreases the chances of injury.

If you are still suffering with an injury, whether tendinitis or some other knee issue, please refer to the exercise program in chapter 4 before embarking on any of these programs. Keep in mind that these programs are not etched in stone, but merely suggestions regarding what you can do to ready your leg for your sport. Please speak to your doctor or other allied health professional before starting any of these routines.

**Soccer**

Soccer is an amazing sport and one of the most popular sports in the world, with a growing number of people around the world interested in playing the "beautiful game." To get your legs in playing-ready shape, here's a routine that can really give you the edge in your power balance and speed. Strong legs create faster and more powerful legs and thus a faster soccer player. What about all that kicking, sprinting, jumping, and passing that you'll be doing on the field? You won't be able to kick a ball very hard without developing strong and balanced legs, especially late in games that move into overtime. Therefore, here are some leg exercises to increase your power, speed, and flexibility on the soccer pitch.

*Exercises*

1. Squats 3 × 10
2. Hack squats 3 × 10
3. Deadlifts 3 × 10

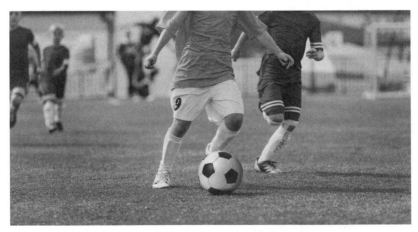

Kids Playing Soccer. *Matimix, image from Bigstockphoto.com*

4. Calf raises 3 × 15–20
5. Bridge 3 × 10
6. Quadriceps stretch 3 × 10 with 30- to 60-second hold
7. Hamstring stretch 3 × 10 with 30- to 60-second hold
8. Hip flexor stretch 3 × 10 with 30- to 60-second hold
9. Balance on one foot, eyes open 3 × 30 seconds
10. Balance on one foot, eyes closed 3 × 30 seconds

Another thing mentioned earlier but that requires a reminder is about the difference in genders when playing soccer. Girls have a higher percentage of knee injuries, most likely ACL and MCL injuries, whereas boys get more muscle strains and ankle injuries. This is due to differences in anatomy. When boys kick a soccer ball, their bodies have a lower center of gravity, causing their knees to bend more, which provides better protection if they get kicked or hit. After puberty, girls develop naturally wider hips and their knees fall inward toward each other, sometimes referred to as "knocked-kneed." On average, their knees also don't bend as much when kicking a ball as boys' knees, leaving them exposed to potential injuries.

The key to limiting injuries in young players lies in a complete warm up. FIFA, the official governing body of soccer around the world, has stated that warm ups using dynamic stretching techniques has reduced injury concerns. The organization has also created programs for females to strengthen their glutes and hamstring muscles to reduce injuries and has even suggested that women should jog backward as well as forward to help strengthen the back part of their body. That is an excellent suggestion for both males and females.

## Skiing

Skiing is a fun sport. Going down your favorite mountain with the wind hitting you as you're making those perfect S lines in the snow is what it's all about. Skiing can also become a difficult and dangerous sport if you don't know what you're doing and you fall because you were flying down the mountain at high speeds. There's not much you can do about pain from injuries resulting from a fall—it comes with the territory—but the most common pain that skiers suffer is at the front of the knee, known as anterior knee pain, and you can do something about that. The most common cause of pain at the front of the knee is patella-femoral joint dysfunction, so here's a sample program that you can do to improve your strength and flexibility.

*Exercises*

1. Inside straight leg raises 3 × 10
2. Inside alphabet ×1
3. Quadriceps stretches 3 × 1 minute
4. Clamshells 3 × 10
5. Deadlifts 3 × 10
6. Bridge 3 × 10
7. Hamstring stretches 3 × 1 minute
8. Step ups 2 × 10–15
9. Squats 3 × 10
10. Calf raises 3 × 15–20

One thing that skiers should work on is their bending at the hips too much. Most skiers tend to "sit down" too much when they ski. This makes it harder for the quads to contract properly and places a ton of stress through the patella-femoral joint and tendons. The best way to prevent this is to train your glutes, especially your gluteus medius and maximus muscles, through the exercises above. Of course, you can try some other exercises, if you like, to get your glutes strong and active. My favorites here are the squats and clamshells. It's beneficial to practice the movement by standing sideways to a mirror and bending your knees so that the weight moves into the front of the feet—not straight down or moving to the back. Try to do about twenty to thirty knee bends using the corrected knee/hip movement a couple of times throughout the day to retrain this movement pattern so that it becomes part of your everyday norms.

## Basketball

Research from the U.S. Consumer Product Safety Commission regarding the types of injuries treated in emergency rooms states that basketball and bicycle injuries sent more Americans to the emergency room than any other types of injuries.

In basketball, there are a lot of stop-and-go motions, as well as cutting maneuvers, which put the ligaments and menisci of the knee at risk.

Injuries to the medial collateral ligaments are most common following a blow to the outside of the knee, and injuries to your anterior cruciate ligament, a more serious injury, happens most often with abrupt changes in direction and landing after jumps. In most cases, a true ACL tear means that your basketball season is over; orthopedic surgery and months of physical therapy are required to get you back on the court the following season.

The most common type of knee strain in basketball is patellar tendonitis, sometimes referred to as jumper's knee. This is an inflammatory condition that causes pain in the front of the knee. Jumper's knee is a very common condition among basketball players because their frequent jumping puts a lot of pressure on the tendons. If you do not have balanced strengthening and stretching programs—not only to get your knee to work properly but also to work in conjunction with your hip and ankle—your NBA career may be cut short.

*Exercises*

1. Inside straight leg raises 3 × 10
2. Inside alphabet × 1
3. Side-lying hip abduction 3 × 10
4. Side-lying hip circles, both directions 2 × 10
5. Leg presses 3 × 10
6. Bridge 3 × 10
7. Clamshells 3 × 10
8. Squats 3 × 10
9. Calf raises 3 × 15–20
10. Deadlifts 3 × 10
11. Quads stretch 3 × 1 minute each leg
12. Hamstring stretch 3 × 1 minute each leg
13. Calf stretch 3 × 1 minute
14. Groin stretch 3 × 1 minute

## Football

Football is America's sport. Millions of kids and grownups play football at every level. It's also one of the sports with the highest number of injuries to the knee area. Injuries normally happen as a result of someone running at full speed then sustaining a full-body tackle. Something's got

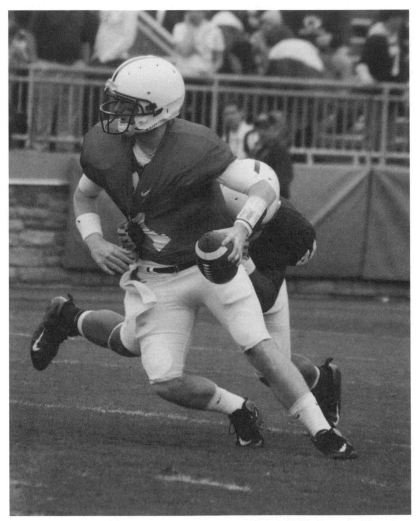

Football. *Finner 1968, image from Bigstockphoto.com*

to give. Knee injuries in football have been shown to be the most frequent, especially those to the ACL or posterior cruciate ligament (PCL) and to the menisci. The medial collateral ligament (MCL) can also become injured when someone hits the outside part of your knee, pushing inward as they tackle you. These types of knee injuries can harm a player's long-term involvement in the sport. Football players also have more knee pulls or sprains due to the surfaces played on and cutting motions at quick speeds.

Strengthening, flexibility, and balance exercises are the best way to keep athletes and weekend warriors healthy and happy.

*Exercises*

1. Deadlifts 3 × 10
2. One-and-a-quarter squats 2 × 10
3. Squats 3 × 10
4. Hamstring curls 3 × 10
5. Clamshells 3 × 10
6. Side-lying hip circles, both directions 3 × 10
7. Quad stretches 3 × 1 minute
8. Hamstring stretches 3 × 1 minute
9. Groin stretches 3 × 1 minute
10. Balance on one foot, eyes open 3 × 30 seconds
11. Balance on one foot, eyes closed 3 × 30 seconds

Wear proper football-style cleats, which have half-inch longer studs than the soccer-style cleats. This type of cleat helps the foot become more mobile. Also, the type of surface that you play on is important. Natural grass is much better than artificial turf, since grass is softer and your knee can absorb more impact than turf. Finally, if you have a preexisting injury and don't feel fully confident about returning to play, wearing a preventative brace helps. Think of it as knee insurance. It will provide the stability that you need to play your game. Use it as a short-term solution until your leg is strong enough to play without it.

## Cycling

Cycling is fun. We all enjoy taking a ride on our bikes and getting fresh air. Others do it competitively. Whether you are an amateur or a pro cyclist, you might have felt a sharp twinge of pain in your knee and probably thought "What just happened?" You're not alone. Knee pain is the most common lower-body problem among us pedal pushers. Most of the times, it's because we push ourselves too much and we don't listen to our body's warning signs. We push ourselves longer or harder than we are physically able to, causing muscle, tendon, or ligament pulls, which can be painful. But what about those stabbing pains that seem to come from nowhere? It might feel like it came out of the blue, but it might be a result of improper equipment or incorrect seat height. It might also be a strength and flexibility imbalance in the legs and hips, which needs to be addressed.

Here's a sample exercise program that should help you ride pain free for a very long time.

*Exercises*

1. Inside straight leg raises 3 × 10
2. Inside alphabet ×1
3. Clamshells 3 × 10
4. Side-lying hip abduction 3 × 10
5. Side-lying hip circles 2 × 10
6. Hamstring curls 3 × 30
7. Deadlifts 3 × 10
8. Prone hip raise knee bending 3 × 10
9. Ab side crunches 3 × 10
10. Quad stretches 3 × 1 minute
11. Hamstring stretches 3 × 1 minute

**At the Office**

We all have busy lives. We want to work out more, but we instead spend a lot of time sitting in front of our desks staring at the computer. Having a relatively inactive lifestyle can cause havoc on our knees. Even worse than not moving our knees is sitting in a position that puts stress on our knees. You might not realize it, but the office environment can be tough on your knees. Sitting down all day and barely moving is not the best thing for our bodies.

Here are some of the bad habits that most of us do without realizing it.

Sitting for six to eight hours a day isn't good for you. If your job calls for you to sit for more than an hour at a time (and most office jobs do), then you'll probably experience knee pain because you're not moving. Your muscles and tendons can become stiff and painful over time. Sitting in the wrong position, like sitting on your feet cross-legged, for long periods can also cause pain by putting pressure on the kneecap.

Also, not sitting in your chair properly can affect your knees. A $500 custom-made chair isn't necessary, but a chair that's in the correct position, at the proper height, with your knees at a 90-degree angle to the floor, and your behind all the way back in the chair rather than perched at the tip can also decrease the stress on your knees.

Here's a sample program that can keep your knees healthy at the office.

*Exercises*

1. One-and-a-quarter squats 3 × 10
2. Clamshells 3 × 10
3. Deadlifts 3 × 10
4. Quadriceps stretch 3 × 1 minute
5. Hamstrings stretch 3 × 1 minute
6. Calf stretch 3 × 1 minute
7. Balance on one foot, eyes open 3 × 30 seconds
8. Balance on one foot, eyes closed 3 × 30 seconds

## SUMMARY

- A balanced strength training and flexibility program is vitally important in reducing knee injuries. It's important to strengthen your weak muscles and stretch your tight ones.
- Squats and deadlift exercises should be the cornerstone of any gym's knee exercise program.
- Keeping the body active by performing a favorite sport is better than sitting at a desk for long hours a day. Consistently moving a little bit every day is much better than sitting for long hours. Your knees, as well as your body, will thank you.

# Notes

## INTRODUCTION

1. K. S. Thomas, K. R. Muir, et al., "Home Based Exercise Programme for Knee Pain and Knee Osteoarthritis: Randomise Controlled Trial, *British Medical Journal*, 325, no. 7367 (2002): 752.

## CHAPTER 2

1. I. Holm and N. Vollestad, "Significant Effect of Gender on Hamstring-to-Quadriceps Strength Ratio and Static Balance in Prepubescent Children from 7 to 12 Years of Age," *American Journal of Sports Medicine* 36, no. 10 (2008): 2007–13.

2. L. A. Zdziarski, Joseph G. Wasser, and Heather K. Vincent, "Chronic Pain Management in the Obese Patient: A Focused Review of Key Challenges and Potential Exercise Solutions," *Journal of Pain Research* 8 (2015): 63–77.

## CHAPTER 3

1. J. C. Segen, *The Dictionary of Modern Medicine* (1992).

2. N. Goldman, M. Chen, T. Fujita, Q. Xu, W. Peng, W. Liu, T. K. Jensen, Y. Pei, F. Wang, X. Han, J.-F. Chen, J. Schnermann, T. Takano, L. Bekar, K. Tieu,

and M. Nedergaard, "Adenosine A1 Receptors Mediate Local Anti-nociceptive Effects of Acupuncture," *Nature Neuroscience* (2010); DOI: 10.1038/nn.2562.


CHAPTER 5


1. E. C. Falvey, R. A. Clark, A. Franklyn-Miller, A. L. Bryant, C. Briggs, and P. R. McCrory, "Iliotibial Band Syndrome: An Examination of the Evidence behind a Number of Treatment Options," *Scandinavian Journal of Medicine and Science in Sports* 20, no. 4 (2010): 580–87.
2. L. J. Distefano, J. T. Blackburn, S. W. Marshall, D. A. Padua, "Gluteal Muscle Activation during Common Therapeutic Exercises," *Journal of Orthopaedic and Sports Physical Therapy* 39, no. 7 (2009): 532–40.


CHAPTER 6


1. B. Jam, "Deep Squatting: Good or Bad?" Advanced Physical Therapy Education Institute, www.aptei.com, 2015.
2. B. Tangtrakulwanich, V. Chongsuvivatwong, and A. F. Geater, "Associations between Floor Activities and Knee Osteoarthritis in Thai Buddhist Monks: The Songkhla Study," *Journal of the Medical Association of Thailand* 89, no. 11 (2006): 1902–8.
3. A. J. Grodzinsky, M. E. Levenston, M. Jin, and E. H. Frank, "Cartilage Tissue Remodeling in Response to Mechanical Forces," *Annual Review of Biomedical Engineering* 2 (2000): 691–713; H. Hartmann, K. Wirth, and M. Klusemann, "Analysis of the Load on the Knee Joint and Vertebral Column with Changes in Squatting Depth and Weight Load," *Sports Medicine* 43, no. 10 (2013): 993–1; B. J. Schoenfeld, "Squatting Kinematics and Kinetics and Their Application to Exercise Performance," *Journal of Strength and Conditioning Research* 24, no. 12 (2010): 3497–506; B. Tangtrakulwanich, V. Chongsuvivatwong, and A. F. Geater, "Associations between Floor Activities and Knee Osteoarthritis in Thai Buddhist Monks: The Songkhla Study," *Journal of the Medical Association of Thailand* 89, no. 11 (2006): 1902–8.
4. Q. T. Nguyen, B. L. Wong, J. Chun, Y. C. Yoon, F. E. Talke, and R. L. Sah, "Macroscopic Assessment of Cartilage Shear: Effects of Counter-Surface Roughness, Synovial Fluid Lubricant, and Compression Offset," *Journal of Biomechanics* 43, no. 9 (2010): 1787–93.

# Bibliography

## CHAPTER 1

Halpern, Brian, and Laura Tucker. *The Knee Crisis Handbook*. Emmaus, PA: Rodale Press, 2003.

Johnson, Jim. *Treat Your Own Knees*. Alameda, CA: Hunter House, 2003.

## CHAPTER 2

DiNubile, Nicholas A. *Framework for the Knee: A 6-Step Plan for Prevention and Injury*. Emmaus, PA: Rodale Press, 2010.

Distefano, L. J., J. T. Blackburn, S. W. Marshall, D. A. Padua. "Gluteal Muscle Activation during Common Therapeutic Exercises." *Journal of Orthopaedic and Sports Physical Therapy* 39, no. 7 (2009): 532–40.

Gilchrist, Julie, Bert R. Mandelbaum, Heidi Melancon, George W. Ryan, Holly J. Silvers, Letha Y. Griffin, Diane S. Watanabe. "A Randomized Controlled Trial to Prevent Noncontact Anterior Cruciate Ligament Injury in Female Collegiate Soccer Players." *American Journal of Sports Medicine* 36, no. 8 (2008).

Holm, I., and N. Vollestad. "Significant Effect of Gender on Hamstring-to-Quadriceps Strength Ratio and Static Balance in Prepubescent Children from 7 to 12 Years of Age." *American Journal of Sports Medicine* 36, no. 10 (2008): 2007–13.

McBeth, J. M., J. E. Earl-Boehm, S. C. Cobb, and W. E. Huddleston. "Hip Muscle Activity during 3 Side-Lying Hip-Strengthening Exercises in Distance Runners." *Journal of Athletic Training* 47, no. 1 (2012): 15–23.

Mountcastle, Sally B., Matthew Posner, John F. Kragh, Dean C. Taylor. "Gender Differences in Anterior Cruciate Ligament Injury Vary with Activity." *American Journal of Sports Medicine* 35, no. 10 (2007).

Presswood, L., J. Cronin, J. W. L. Keogh, C. Whatman. "Gluteus Medius: Applied Anatomy, Dysfunction, Assessment, and Progressive Strengthening." *Strength and Conditioning Journal* 30, no. 5 (2008): 41–53.

Soballe, K., and P. Kjaersgaard-Andersen. "Ruptured Tibialis Posterior Tendon in a Closed Ankle Fracture." *Clinical Orthopaedics and Related Research* 231 (1988): 140–43.

Zdziarski, L. A., Joseph G. Wasser, and Heather K. Vincent. "Chronic Pain Management in the Obese Patient: A Focused Review of Key Challenges and Potential Exercise Solutions." *Journal of Pain Research* 8 (2015): 63–77.

## CHAPTER 3

Andrews, J. "Supplements That Rebuild Collagen." Accessed 29 January 2012. www.livestrong.com/article/357927-supplements-that-re-buildcollagen.

DiNubile, Nicholas A. *Framework for the Knee: A 6-Step Plan for Prevention and Injury.* Emmaus, PA: Rodale Press, 2010.

Goldman, Nanna, Michael Chen, Takumi Fujita, Qiwu Xu, Weiguo Peng, Wei Liu, Tina K. Jensen, Yong Pei, Fushun Wang, Xiaoning Han, Jiang-Fan Chen, Jurgen Schnermann, Takahiro Takano, Lane Bekar, Kim Tieu, and Maiken Nedergaard. "Adenosine A1 Receptors Mediate Local Anti-Nociceptive Effects of Acupuncture." *Nature Neuroscience* (2010); DOI: 10.1038/nn.2562.

Segen, J. C. *The Dictionary of Modern Medicine.* Park Ridge, NJ: Parthenon Publishing Group, 1992.

Speed, C. "Shoulder Pain." Accessed February 2006. Online version of *BMJ Clinical Evidence.*

## CHAPTER 4

Daneshjoo, A., A. H. Mokhtar, N. Rahnama, A. Yusof. "The Effects of Injury Preventive Warm-up Programs on Knee Strength Ratio in Young Male Professional Soccer Players." *PLOS ONE* 7, no. 12 (2012), DOI: 10.1371/journal.pone.0050979.

## CHAPTER 5

Falvey, E. C., R. A. Clark, A. Franklyn-Miller, A. L. Bryant, C. Briggs, and P. R. McCrory. "Iliotibial Band Syndrome: An Examination of the Evidence behind a Number of Treatment Options." *Scandinavian Journal of Medicine and Science in Sports* 20, no. 4 (2010): 580–87.

Moore, K. L. *Clinically Oriented Anatomy*. Baltimore: Williams and Wilkins, 1985.

Soballe, K., and P. Kjaersgaard-Andersen. "Ruptured Tibialis Posterior Tendon in a Closed Ankle Fracture." *Clinical Orthopaedics and Related Research* 231 (1988): 140–43.

Starrett, K. *Ready to Run*. Las Vegas, NV: Victory Belt Publishing, 2014.

Travell, J. G., and D. G. Simons. *Myofascial Pain and Dysfunction: The Trigger Point Manual for the Lower Extremities*. Baltimore: Williams and Wilkins, 1992.


## CHAPTER 6

Farley, K. "Analysis of the Conventional Deadlift." *Strength and Conditioning Journal* 17, no. 6 (1995): 55–57.

Grodzinsky, A. J., M. E. Levenston, M. Jin, and E. H. Frank. "Cartilage Tissue Remodeling in Response to Mechanical Forces." *Annual Review of Biomedical Engineering* 2 (2000): 691–713.

Hartmann, H., K. Wirth, and M. Klusemann. "Analysis of the Load on the Knee Joint and Vertebral Column with Changes in Squatting Depth and Weight Load." *Sports Medicine* 43, no. 10 (2013): 993–1008.

Nguyen, Q. T., B. L. Wong, J. Chun, Y. C. Yoon, F. E. Talke, and R. L. Sah. "Macroscopic Assessment of Cartilage Shear: Effects of Counter-Surface Roughness, Synovial Fluid Lubricant, and Compression Offset." *Journal of Biomechanics* 43, no. 9 (2010): 1787–93.

Schoenfeld, B. J. "Squatting Kinematics and Kinetics and Their Application to Exercise Performance." *Journal of Strength and Conditioning Research* 24, no. 12 (2010): 3497–506.

Tangtrakulwanich, B., V. Chongsuvivatwong, and A. F. Geater. "Associations between Floor Activities and Knee Osteoarthritis in Thai Buddhist Monks: The Songkhla Study." *Journal of the Medical Association of Thailand* 89, no. 11 (2006): 1902–8.

Wright, G. A., T. H. Delong, and G. Gehlsen. "Electromyographic Activity of the Hamstrings during Performance of the Leg Curl, Stiff-leg Deadlift, and Back Squat Movements." *The Journal of Strength and Conditioning Research* 13, no. 2 (1999): 168–74.

# Index